The Heart

Its Function in Health and Disease

PERSPECTIVES IN MEDICINE
Leo van der Reis, M.D., General Editor

Selzer   *The Heart: Its Function in Health and Disease*

The Heart

Its Function in Health and Disease

ARTHUR SELZER, M.D.

UNIVERSITY OF CALIFORNIA PRESS

Berkeley and Los Angeles   1966

University of California Press
Berkeley and Los Angeles, California

Cambridge University Press
London, England

© 1966 by The Regents of the University of California
Library of Congress Catalog Card Number: 65-25023

Designed by Adrian Wilson

Printed in the United States of America

Editor's Foreword

During the last decade, general public interest in medicine has greatly increased. Today there is a real need for reliable and intelligible information about developments in the science and art of medicine. A wide gap exists between technical scientific papers in the journals and popular—and sometimes erroneous or misleading—accounts written for a mass audience.

This new series of books is intended for serious readers who wish to learn more about current medicine but who cannot and should not be expected to read textbooks or scientific journals intended for physicians and medical students. Our intention is to present the fundamentals of each subject in terminology that is understandable to the educated reader who is not trained in medicine. We hope, also, that the volumes will be useful to students in the biological sciences and to those whose work brings them into contact with medical issues: social workers, jurists, pharmacists, psychologists, and others. Perhaps, too, the practicing physician will find help in formulating answers to the questions of his patients, since a better understanding of diseases and of bodily functions can dispel fears and superstitions that sometimes delay or hamper treatment. If some of these purposes are served, the books will justify the time and effort expended by the authors.

Each book will be a concise, comprehensive, and illustrated essay on a major disease, or a body system and its fundamentally related parts, or a specialized area of research, or an aspect of our society that affects the public health. Historical and sociological factors will be included where appropriate.

LEO VAN DER REIS, M.D.
General Editor

Preface

The invitation to participate in the series, "Perspectives in Medicine," was a welcome challenge to me. It is, indeed, fitting that the opening work of this series should be devoted to diseases of the heart and blood vessels, which constitute the foremost medical problem in the country today. More than one-half of all deaths in the United States are caused directly or indirectly by diseases of the heart and blood vessels. A recent survey conducted by the United States Public Health Service showed that an estimated 14.6 million out of 111 million adult Americans (one-eighth of the total) have some form of heart disease, and another eighth is suspected of having heart disease. The great concern with this staggering problem is shown by two events which took place in the fall of 1964: In November some 500 experts met in Washington as the Second National Conference on Cardiovascular Diseases in order to review the accomplishments of the past fifteen years and to make plans for the future. About the same time the President's Commission on Heart Disease, Cancer and Stroke published its report, entitled "A National Program to Conquer Heart Disease, Cancer and Stroke."

It is evident to all concerned with the problem of heart disease that new knowledge is greatly needed and that new developments in the field of diagnosis and treatment should be made available as rapidly as possible to as many patients as possible. Thus research in heart disease is being conducted in virtually every important medical center. It ranges from basic laboratory studies by biochemists and biophysicists to health surveys and observations of entire communities. Large sums of money are expended for heart research by the National Heart Institute (a branch of the U. S. Public Health Service) and by the American Heart Association and its chapters. Other voluntary agencies and foundations also contribute significant sums to heart research. However, the problem of heart disease transcends heart research and its application in diagnosis and treatment; it has a broad economic impact upon our society, for it includes such aspects as employability of individuals with heart disease, their rehabilitation and retraining, vocational guidance and work classification of employable cardiacs, and, perhaps most important, the economic impact of heart disease upon the patient and his family. The precise diagnostic methods and surgical treatments now available for certain forms of heart disease require expensive equipment and skilled teams of experts, which are often beyond the means of the average family. Various forms of health insurance as well as such governmental agencies as the U. S. Children's Bureau, the U. S. Office of Vocational Rehabilitation, and state agencies for crippled children provide welcome assistance to those suffering heart ailments, but many individuals still face financial hardship when afflicted with heart disease—a fact acknowledged in the recommendations of the President's Commission that deal with the creation of regional centers for the diagnosis and treatment of heart disease.

The subject of health and disease is of interest to every individual. The enlightened public of today demands much more detailed information concerning health matters than did the public of a generation ago. In the field of heart disease many books written for laymen are already available as well as the many excellent publications sponsored by the American Heart Association. These publications serve primarily as sources of information for the patient with heart disease and for his family in implementing the physician's recommendations and aiding in the doctor-patient relationship. Readers interested in the more scientific aspects of heart disease are kept informed by science writers' accounts of recent advances in this field. Many such articles are of high scientific and literary caliber and contain accurate scientific information. However, such writings are of necessity slanted toward the new, dramatic, spectacular, and often still experimental aspects of heart research and can provide neither a complete nor a balanced picture. It is the objective of this book to provide the reader with a systematic, clear presentation of current views in the field of diseases of the heart and blood vessels told in a conservative and objective manner. It is hoped that this book will fill the gap between "popular" publications and books written for those with a medical background. It is felt that such a book should be written in technical terms, but all of them are defined in the text and most are included in the glossary for ready reference. It is also hoped that the exposition will be comprehensible to all who have a basic knowledge of high school physics and biology. If these objectives are fulfilled and the book advances public understanding of a complex and vital area of medicine today, I will be more than gratified.

ARTHUR SELZER, M.D.

San Francisco
July, 1965

Contents

Part One

Introduction

1

The Heart and Circulation: Yesterday, Today, and Tomorrow

The pre-Christian Greek philosophers recognized that the heart was of key importance in the human body. The structure of the heart and its relationship to the blood vessels were fairly well understood by Hippocrates, Aristotle, Erasistratus, and others. However, the role of the heart in the circulation of the blood was not clearly set forth until many centuries later. Indeed, an erroneous description originating with Galen of Pergamon (A.D. 138-201) was accepted as correct for hundreds of years, confusing students and practitioners of medicine alike. Galen postulated that blood was formed in the liver from ingested food and then flowed to the right side of the heart. From there he thought that part of the blood went to the lungs and part was transported through invisible "pores" in the septum to the left ventricle, where it mixed with "vital spirits"—the air inhaled in the lungs. Galen and his followers also believed that the blood ebbed to and fro in the arteries supplying the various organs. Despite their fallacious interpretation of heart function, Galen and his disciples did point out that the heart was subject to disease. This belief was in contrast to the teachings of the earlier philosophers, who considered that the organ was immune to disease. Galen also demonstrated that the blood vessels contain blood and not air, as the Alexandrian school of medicine had been teaching for over four hundred years.

3

During the Renaissance, definite advances were made in the knowledge of the heart and circulation. Dissection of the cardiovascular system in humans permitted fairly accurate descriptions of the structure of the heart and blood vessels in health and disease. Excellent drawings were made by Leonardo da Vinci (1452-1519) and by the famous anatomist Andreas Vesalius (1514-1564). But it was not until 1628 that the correct functioning of the circulatory system was formulated. This was in the monumental *De motu cordis* (*On the Motion of the Heart*) by Harvey.

William Harvey (1578-1657) was one of the giants of medical science. Educated at Cambridge and at Padua—then the most famous medical center in Europe—Harvey was a prominent teacher and practitioner of medicine in London. He became intrigued by the seeming discrepancies between the actual structure of the heart and blood vessels and the existing theory of blood circulation. Harvey set out to discover the true sequence of the flow of blood. He did so by a combination of brilliant deductions and carefully designed experiments. First, he discarded the Galenian concepts of "invisible pores" in the septum as well as that of the flow of blood back and forth in the vessels. He also rejected the idea that the two ventricles had different functions; noting their identical structure, he deduced that they must also have identical functions—the propelling of blood into two circuits. He surmised that if each ventricle were to eject even one or two ounces of blood per heartbeat, the quantity of blood ejected in an hour would be many times greater than the total quantity of blood in the body; hence, blood must move in a *circle*. Harvey performed a series of experiments designed to stop the circulation of blood by placing ligatures on various blood vessels and observing the direction of blood flow in the superficial veins of the human arm (fig. 1). From these experiments he correctly outlined the path of the circulation. His treatise *De motu cordis* contains a complete and accurate description of the circulation of blood concisely presented in seventeen short chapters—a masterpiece of exposition.

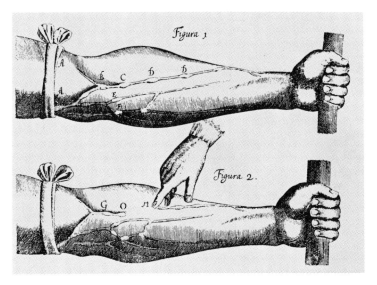

FIGURE 1. *Reproduction of one of the illustrations from Harvey's* De motu cordis, *showing his experiment establishing the direction of blood flow in the veins of the human arm by observing the superficial veins after placing a tourniquet on the arm.*

During the eighteenth century many ideas concerning the structure and function of the heart and circulation were crystallized; at the same time great strides were made in understanding the nature of heart diseases, and in diagnosing and treating them. Among the noteworthy accomplishments of this period were the physiological studies by the Reverend Stephen Hales (1677-1761), whose principal interest, however, was in plant physiology. He performed the first experiment designed to measure the pressure and velocity of blood flow in animals. He placed a glass tube—the first manometer—in the artery of the neck of a horse and by measuring the height of the column of blood (7½ feet) he determined its pressure (fig. 2), thus making the first measurement of "blood pressure."

William Heberden (1710-1801), a fashionable London phy-

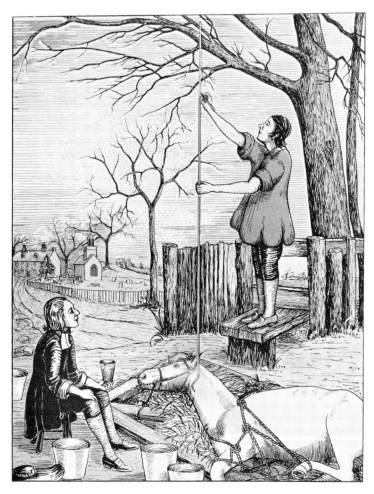

FIGURE 2. *The first measurement of blood pressure by the Reverend Stephen Hales, who with the aid of an assistant placed a glass tube in the neck artery of a horse and observed the blood rise in the tube to a height of 7 1/2 feet. (Reproduced by permission of* Medical Times*)*

sician, among whose patients was Dr. Samuel Johnson, gave a vivid and accurate description of chest pain related to heart disease. He described in great detail all the features of what he termed "pectoris dolor" (chest pain), from which the still currently used phrase "angina pectoris" is derived. He so well described the features of this type of pain that his description could be included in a present-day textbook. Yet Heberden was unaware of the true nature of this symptom, considering it a "spasmodic" disorder. Heberden's contemporary, John Hunter (1729-1793), a famous London physician and surgeon who first designed an operation for treatment of an aneurysm (abnormal swelling of a blood vessel), himself suffered from angina pectoris during the last seven years of his life. He was well aware of the seriousness of his condition and of the role of excitement in producing this type of chest pain. Hunter made the oft-quoted statement, "My life is in the hands of any rascal who chooses to annoy and tease me," which turned out to be prophetic, for he died after a violent argument with his colleagues at a meeting in St. George's Hospital in London. Edward Jenner (1749-1823), the father of smallpox vaccine, was aware of the connection between Hunter's type of chest pain and abnormalities of the coronary arteries. He correctly predicted that such diseased coronary arteries would be found in John Hunter's heart.

Another fascinating episode in the history of cardiology was the discovery of digitalis, still today the most important drug in the treatment of heart disease. William Withering (1741-1799), a practitioner of medicine whose hobby was botany, became interested in the fact that an old woman in his native Shropshire successfully used a herb tea to relieve dropsy, which physicians were helpless in treating. As a botanist, it was easy for him to demonstrate that the active ingredient of the tea was foxglove. Withering began using foxglove in his own practice, proving its value. While he was not fully aware that foxglove is primarily active in "dropsy" caused by heart disease, and used it for all types of body swelling, he did observe that foxglove had some action upon the heart by slowing the pulse rate. He told of his experiences in the classic *An Account of the Foxglove,* which even by modern standards is an excellent treatise on the action, use, and toxicity of digitalis.

Early in the nineteenth century the Frenchman René Laënnec (1781-1826) invented the stethoscope. At the time the technique of auscultation (listening to heart sounds) was rarely used but, when used, required the physician to place his ear directly upon the patient's chest. Laënnec describes vividly his discovery in his famous book *De l'auscultation mediate* (*Treatise on Mediate Auscultation*). He wrote that in 1816 he was asked to see a plump young woman suspected of having heart disease. Because of her obesity the standard techniques of palpation and percussion of the heart were useless. He wished to try auscultation, but propriety prevented him from placing his ear upon the patient's chest. He then recalled a simple fact in acoustics, the transmission and augmentation of sound through certain solid bodies, such as the scratch of a pin at one end of a piece of wood heard while applying the other end to one's ear. He rolled a piece of paper into a cylinder and to his delight found that he could hear the young woman's "heart action" even better than by direct auscultation. Laënnec then designed a wooden stethoscope, cylindrical in shape (fig. 3). Laënnec's discovery had a tremendous impact upon progress in diagnosis of heart disease, but, as often happens, he received no recognition from his close associates. Not until his book made him world-famous and physicians from all over Europe began traveling to Paris to attend his ward at the Necker Hospital was he advanced to professorship at the Collège de France and membership in the French Academy of Medicine. Laënnec's principal interest centered around diseases of the lungs. His book, *A Treatise on the Diseases of the Chest,* contains chapters dealing with diseases of the heart which, unfortunately, had many errors. These, however, were corrected by his disciples in later editions.

During the second half of the nineteenth century great strides toward correct diagnosis of heart disease were made. The era was dominated by the pathologists, who established gross and

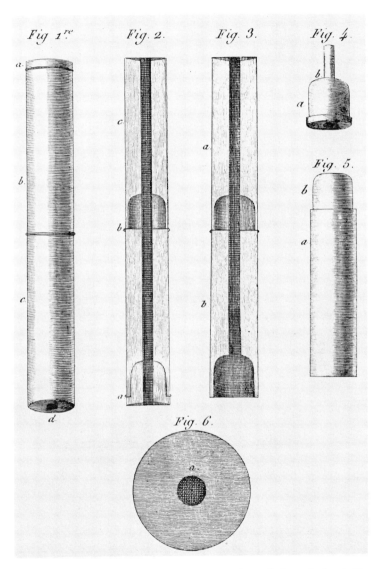

FIGURE 3. *Reproduction of the illustration from Laënnec's book* De l'auscultation mediate, *showing the details of the construction of his wooden stethoscope. Laënnec provided a description of the components and added, "Any turner will be able to make the instrument from the above description."*

microscopic criteria for diseases of the heart and circulation. The goal of the physicians was to diagnose structural abnormalities of the heart, and they paid little attention to functions of the heart and circulation. And yet the astuteness of the diagnosticians was indeed remarkable, considering that their work was based entirely upon physical examination and that their only available instrument was Laënnec's wooden stethoscope. The world-famous medical center in Vienna was then dominated by two great men, both Czechs: Carl Rokitansky (1804-1878) and Joseph Skoda (1805-1881). Rokitansky was a pathologist whose principal interest was diseases of the heart. He described and classified some of the most complex congenital malformations of the heart. Skoda built his reputation as the most famous diagnostician in Europe. Yet his brilliance in diagnosis was matched by his discouragement with the available means of treatment of chronic diseases. Skoda's therapeutic nihilism was as famous as his diagnostic skill. The state of medicine (particularly cardiology) in that era is best illustrated by the irreverent saying that "patients from all over the world came to Vienna to have the diagnosis made by Skoda and to have it proved correct by Rokitansky—at autopsy."

At the same time as clinicians were establishing the background for modern diagnosis of heart disease, physiologists were busy studying fundamentals of the functions of the heart and circulation. The physiology of the circulatory system was thoroughly investigated in animal laboratories, particularly in France and Germany.

At the turn of the last century clinical cardiology and cardiovascular physiology were totally separated from each other. The physician was concerned with diseases, which he saw only from the standpoint of alteration in structure. The physiologist, working entirely on animals, was concerned with the study of normal function and had practically no opportunity to study abnormal function related to disease. The great change came when various instrumental methods were designed which permitted the study of certain functions in man. The introduction of physiological thinking to clinical cardiology brought a third dimension into cardiology, and the modern era of comprehension of heart disease began. The earliest clinical instruments included the mercury manometer for measuring blood pressure, the polygraph for the correlative study of human pulses, and the electrocardiograph. In order to measure arterial blood pressure, the mercury manometer was adapted for use in humans by Scipione Riva Rocci, an Italian physiologist. His apparatus, reported in 1896, was the prototype of the modern "blood pressure cuff." The polygraph was an instrument designed by Sir James Mackenzie, who in 1908 adapted a large pulse-recording device using smoked drums into a small portable instrument using ink and paper. The electrocardiograph was developed by William Einthoven in Holland in 1906.

The first disorder of the heart function to undergo thorough investigation by clinicians was disturbances of rhythm of the heart, or arrhythmias. This field was so completely investigated that most of the concepts developed during these early studies are fully valid today. Among the contributors to the early physiological studies in human heart disease three names occupy prominent places: Sir James Mackenzie (1853-1925), Sir Thomas Lewis (1881-1945), and Professor Karel Frederik Wenckebach (1864-1940). Mackenzie, a Scotsman who practiced medicine in the small English town of Burnley in Lancashire, became interested in disturbances of heart rhythm and made observations on his private patients. He designed the polygraph in his spare time, and by astute observations laid the foundation for the modern concepts of arrhythmias. At the age of 54, already a world-famous author of books and articles, Mackenzie was induced to give up country practice. He moved to London and devoted himself to a consulting practice in cardiology and to teaching. Lewis, a Welshman working in London, was a pupil of Mackenzie who expounded his teacher's theories and investigated them further in animals and in humans with the use of the electrocardiograph. Lewis was probably the most important pioneer in the field of clinical physiology (called by him "clinical science"), which is the bedside study of heart function in patients, using physiological methods—a branch of cardiology which only recently has become widely popular. Wenckebach, a Dutchman who became professor of medicine in Vienna, was one of the last "greats" in this former Mecca of clinical medicine. He made many important contributions to the knowledge of arrhythmias, among them the use of quinine and its derivative, quinidine, in the treatment of disturbances of heart rhythm. Wenckebach's attention was drawn to quinine by one of his patients, a merchant from the Dutch East Indies, who suffered from palpitations (atrial fibrillation) and observed that whenever he took quinine for the prevention of malaria his attacks disappeared. Alerted, Wenckebach investigated quinine and, noting its weak action, encouraged his pupil, W. Frey, to study other extracts from the bark of the cinchona tree. These studies led to the isolation of quinidine, a highly effective cardiac drug.

In the United States, James Herrick of Chicago (1861-1954) recognized a special form of cardiac pain (angina pectoris), one of unusually long duration, which he correctly identified as being caused by coronary occlusion (obstruction). His classic paper, published in 1912, made very little impact upon the medical profession for about fifteen years, until it became obvious that coronary occlusion indeed constitutes a common and important variety of "heart attack."

The period between World War I and II saw important developments in many areas of cardiology. For the first time meaningful treatment of heart disease became possible: proper methods for administrating digitalis were developed; the cardiac use of quinidine became widely known; and new and powerful diuretic drugs were introduced. The electrocardiograph and the X ray came into general use, and their value in the diagnosis of many forms of heart disease was recognized. Finally, pioneering work in the field of cardiovascular surgery proved the feasibility of surgical treatment of some forms of cardiovascular disease.

Clinical cardiology in the United States was dominated largely by the Boston school, because of the impact of three personalities: Paul Dudley White (1886-), Samuel A. Levine (1891-), and Soma Weiss (1899-1941). White has made numerous contributions to the field of clinical cardiology. His scholarly book *Heart Disease* has become a classic; in it he incorporated the modern classifications of heart disease, largely developed by himself and by Richard Cabot. Levine, among whose many contributions are the first major monograph on coronary thrombosis and a popular book, *Clinical Heart Disease,* became particularly well known as an astute diagnostician. White and Levine, today's deans of cardiology, have among their pupils many prominent cardiologists all over the world. Weiss, whose tragically premature death was a major loss to cardiology, was a pioneer in the field of clinical physiology, his work proceeding along lines similar to those of Thomas Lewis in England.

However, it was during World War II that knowledge of cardiology expanded so greatly that it brought about a major reorientation of thinking. It has been said with much justification that recent progress in this field in ten years surpassed all previous advances in the entire history of cardiology! Accomplishments of the years since World War II are far too numerous to describe, and one can merely mention the over-all trends.

New and precise research methods in biochemistry and physiology have brought about a better understanding of heart disease. Clinical physiology and clinical biochemistry become important branches of medicine. The impact of the study of physiological functions and biochemical processes penetrated not only into the scholarly atmosphere of the medical school center but into the everyday practice of cardiology, making clinical cardiology more of a science than an empirical art, as it had been in the past. The development of such methods as cardiac catheterization and angiocardiography (see Glossary) not only opened the doors to new and fascinating studies of disease in man but also immensely increased the precision of diagnostic work.

Rapid progress in the field of cardiovascular surgery has permitted the curing and correcting of an ever-increasing number

of heart diseases, providing at the same time splendid opportunities to study many aspects of human physiology.

New developments in medical treatment (antibiotics, drugs
for the control of hypertension) have favorably affected the
course of some forms of heart disease previously considered
either incurable or uncontrollable.

The beginning of emphasis upon preventive aspects of heart
disease has stimulated research at international levels and has
laid the groundwork for a broad epidemiological approach to the
problem of heart disease.

Today's cardiology is obviously dominated by the more spectacular aspects of treatment of heart disease. The almost miraculous results of open-heart surgery, the advances of vascular
surgery, the electronic control of the heartbeat, the introduction
of powerful new drugs—all these have made the field of cardiovascular disease one of the most exciting in medicine today both
for the physician and the layman. And yet, away from the limelight, are the scientists working quietly in their laboratories on
the problems still unsolved. They are the men who investigate
the microstructure of heart muscle cells, the biochemical aspects
of cell metabolism, the genetic code of cells, and many other
aspects of basic physiology and biochemistry. It may be many
years before discoveries in these basic fields can be translated
into practical advances, and yet the growing understanding of
the basic facts of nature is one of the most challenging aspects
of today's scientific world.

Where is cardiology heading? It is virtually certain that progress will continue along present lines: more effective drugs for
control of various aspects of heart disease will be found; better
and safer operations will be available; further refinements in
diagnosis will be made; and many processes will be better understood. But we must look beyond these advances to the broader
aspects of heart disease. Two fundamental questions will have to
be answered: (1) Can heart disease be effectively prevented and
therefore totally eliminated? and (2) Is the "ultimate" in treatment possible: replacement of the diseased heart by a mechani-

cal heart or by a transplanted healthy heart? Extensive research into the causes of atherosclerosis, hypertension, and birth defects has not even begun to provide an understanding of the problem, and a thorough understanding is necessary before one can consider whether such diseases are preventable. The problem of total heart replacement is at a point where the difficulties are seemingly insurmountable, contrary to the totally unrealistic statements made to the public from time to time that such developments are "just around the corner." Nevertheless, one cannot help recalling that only two decades ago operating on the open heart or replacing diseased valves with artificial ones seemed fantastically improbable.

2

The Normal Heart and Circulation: Structure

The heart is a remarkable organ indeed. Entrusted with the task of distributing blood throughout the body, it contracts and relaxes about 100,000 times in 24 hours and pumps more than 2,000 gallons of blood during that time. Called upon to work continuously, even during sleep, the heart knows no rest other than the brief period of relaxation, less than half a second, between each pumping action. In order to perform its job—to contract nearly half a billion times during a lifetime—its structure consists of the most rugged muscle in the body and has many work-saving devices. The essential part of the heart is its muscle, which envelops the cavity filled with blood and which has the shape of a cone, so that a relatively small foreshortening of the muscle ejects the blood with considerable force. The directional flow of blood is regulated by effective one-way valves.

The circulatory system consists of a series of tubes in which blood is propelled throughout the body. Arteries, vessels directing the flow from the heart toward the various organs, have thick walls endowed with considerable elasticity, a feature that saves the pumping work of the heart by cushioning the high pressure generated during contraction of the heart and the fall in pressure expected to take place during its relaxation. The microscopically thin capillaries are permeable to vital substances; they are contained in the various tissues and organs of the body and constitute the final destination of the circulatory system. The circle is com-

16

*pleted by the channels bringing the blood back to the heart. These
blood vessels, the veins, are thin-walled; the blood flows in them
in a leisurely fashion, under low pressure, its flow facilitated by the
motion of muscles.*

GENERAL DEFINITIONS

The circulatory apparatus is a closed system filled with blood,
consisting of the heart and blood vessels; it is the principal supply line between various organs and parts of the body. The
circulation delivers "fuel" to the body, namely oxygen and other
essential substances; it also removes carbon dioxide and other
products of metabolism. Blood is circulated in two separate circuits: the smaller circuit is referred to as the *lesser circulation* or
the *pulmonary circulation;* and the larger circuit, the *greater
circulation* or the *systemic circulation.* The former supplies the
lungs, the latter all other organs of the body. Figure 4 is a diagrammatic outline of the circulation, showing the pulmonary
circulation above the heart and the greater circulation below the
heart.

The central organ of the circulatory system is the *heart.* It consists of two separate pumps, one for each circuit, simultaneously
ejecting an equal quantity of blood into the greater and the lesser
circulation. The heart is a muscular organ weighing approximately 300 gm., which contracts rhythmically about 70 times a
minute, and with each beat expels about 75 cc. of blood into
each circuit. Each system of blood vessels into which the blood
is pumped consists of three parts: the *arterial system,* the *capillary system,* and the *venous system,* as shown in figure 4. The
objective of the lesser circulation is to send blood through the
vessels of the lungs and there to bring it into close contact with
the air, so that oxygen can be replenished and carbon dioxide
removed. Thus the blood in the pulmonary artery (leading to
the lungs) has a low oxygen content and high carbon dioxide
content, whereas blood returning from the lungs in the pulmonary veins has a high oxygen content and low carbon dioxide

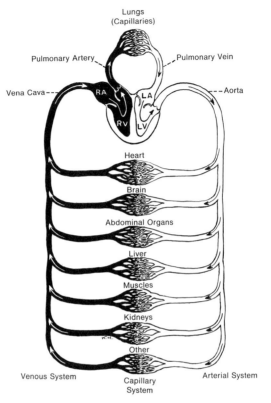

Lungs
(Capillaries)

Pulmonary Artery

Pulmonary Vein

Vena Cava

RA

LA

Aorta

RV

LV

Heart

Brain

Abdominal Organs

Liver

Muscles

Kidneys

Other

Venous System

Capillary
System

Arterial System

FIGURE 4. *General diagram of the circulation, showing the pulmonary circuit above the heart and the systemic circuit below the heart. Oxygenated blood is shown white and de-oxygenated (venous) blood black.*

content. The objectives of the greater circulation are as follows: to deliver oxygen to the tissues; to pick up and deliver all nourishing substances, vitamins, hormones, and other vital compounds; to carry carbon dioxide, the "exhaust" of the tissues, to the right side of the heart and hence to the lungs for elimination; and to pick up other waste products and deliver them to the points of their excretion or elimination (kidneys, liver, etc.).

Oxygen is the most essential fuel for every tissue of the body.

Its utilization is intimately connected with carbon dioxide, the principal waste product of tissues. Thus, each cell in the body "breathes" by extracting oxygen from the blood and by depositing carbon dioxide in its place. Blood destined *for* the tissues, fully saturated with oxygen and containing a lower quantity of carbon dioxide, is bright red. It is ordinarily referred to as *arterial blood,* as it is contained in the arteries of the greater circulation. Blood returning *from* the tissues has a lower oxygen content and is high in carbon dioxide; such blood, dark red in color, is termed *venous blood,* as it is contained in the veins of the systemic circulation. It shines through the superficial veins under the skin, giving them the appearance of being blue. It is clear from figure 4 that the terms "arterial blood" (indicated as white in the chart) and "venous blood" (indicated as black) apply only to the greater circulation. In the pulmonary circulation, as we have said, the role of arteries and veins is reversed. Figure 4 emphasizes the fact that the pulmonary circuit consists of a simple system of vessels supplying a single organ; the greater circulation, on the other hand, consists of a great number of semiautonomous systems connected parallel to each other. Each organ of the body receives blood from arterial branches, which then divide into capillary branches. The actual exchange of all substances between the blood and tissues occurs within the capillary system.

STRUCTURE OF THE HEART

The heart is a muscular, conical organ located in the center of the chest, slightly more to the left than to the right (fig. 5). It has an apex, directed downward and leftward, and a base at its upper part where major vessels originate. The heart consists of three layers: an inner lining (*endocardium*); the heart muscle (*myocardium*); and the outer lining (*pericardium*). The pericardium actually has two layers: the outer layer of the heart, which is firmly attached to it (*epicardium*), giving the surface of the heart a smooth, glistening appearance; and another layer (*parietal pericardium*), which constitutes a loose sack in which the heart

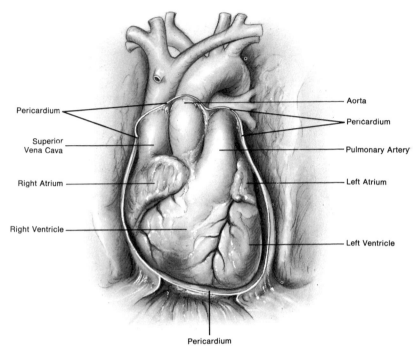

Pericardium

Aorta

Pericardium

Superior Vena Cava

Pulmonary Artery

Right Atrium

Left Atrium

Right Ventricle

Left Ventricle

Pericardium

FIGURE 5. *Appearance of the front aspect of the heart with the parietal pericardium removed.*

is suspended. This parietal pericardium is shown in figure 5, where the front portion of it has been removed in order to show details of the frontal aspect of the heart. Between the two layers of the pericardium there is a small amount of fluid (*pericardial fluid*) which acts as a lubricant, facilitating motion of the heart within the pericardiac sac.

The heart is a hollow organ which consists of four chambers: two *atria* (the correct term "atrium" is often used interchangeably with the older term "auricle") and two *ventricles*. The thin-walled atria act as receptacles for the blood returning to the heart; the thick-walled ventricles, consisting of several layers of muscle, constitute the pump proper. The two atria and the two ventricles are separated from each other by partitions called *septums*. As mentioned, the heart is a twin pump: the right side of the heart (right atrium and right ventricle) handles venous blood; the left side of the heart (left atrium and left ventricle) handles arterial blood. The independent function of the two sides of the heart is often acknowledged by referring to them as the "right heart" and the "left heart." The respective locations of the four chambers, as they appear when looking at the front surface of the heart, are shown in figure 5.

Venous blood enters the *right atrium* through two large veins and a small vein. The large veins, *superior vena cava* and *inferior vena cava,* channel blood from the upper and lower parts of the body, respectively. The third channel, the *coronary sinus,* delivers venous blood from the heart itself. The right atrium and its three tributary channels are shown in figure 6. The right atrium is an irregularly shaped chamber connecting, by way of a large opening, with the right ventricle This orifice is protected by the *tricuspid valve.* The two large veins enter the atrium at its upper and lower right portions, respectively. The coronary sinus empties itself into the right atrium at its lower back wall. The mixture of blood derived from the three channels flows into the right ventricle through the tricuspid orifice. The right ventricle is

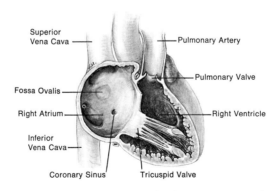

FIGURE 6. *Right side of the heart shown with its front wall removed. Description in text.*

usually divided into two portions: the lower portion, the inflow tract (behind the tricuspid valve); and the upper portion, the outflow tract, leading to the pulmonary orifice. At the top of the conical outflow tract is the pulmonary artery, separated from the tract by the outflow valve of the right side of the heart—the pulmonary valve. The contents of the right ventricle are ejected into the pulmonary artery, destined for the lungs.

The left side of the heart is almost identical in structure with the right side. The left atrium contains the orifices of four pulmonary veins, two of which drain blood from each lung. This atrium is located on the posterior (back) part of the heart; the pulmonary veins enter on its posterior surface. Its lower part is open, leading into the left ventricle. The connecting opening, the *mitral orifice*, contains the *mitral valve*. The left ventricle has a relatively small, conical cavity. The muscle of the left ventricle is three or four times thicker than that of the right ventricle. This relationship is in line with differences in pressure between the two sides of the heart. The upper part of the left ventricle contains both orifices: the inflow (mitral) orifice, to the left and rear, and the outflow (aortic orifice) in front and to the right. The aorta originates from the left ventricle in a manner similar to that of the pulmonary artery from the right. Its origin contains the aortic valve.

As indicated, the two sides of the heart are separated from each other by partitions (*septums*): the atrial septum, and the ventricular septum. The former consists of a thin layer of muscle, with the exception of an oval area where muscle is missing—the *fossa ovalis* (fig. 6). This is a remnant of a valve, present in the embryo, which protected an orifice between the two atria through which blood could flow from the right atrium into the left atrium before birth (see chap. 13). The ventricular septum consists of a thick muscle continuous with the "free" walls of the left ventricle. It is thinned out in only one small area, underneath the aortic valves, where no muscle is present (*membranous septum*). This is a common site of birth defects in which this portion of the septum is missing, providing a communication between the two ventricles (see fig. 29).

The four heart *valves* consist of two sets almost identical in structure and function. The two inflow valves separate the atria from the ventricles (*atrioventricular valves*). The outflow valves separate the ventricles from the two main arterial trunks (*semilunar valves*). The inflow valves prevent blood from backing into the atria during ventricular contraction and ejection of the blood into the arterial trunks. The purpose of the semilunar valves is to prevent the sucking back of blood from the aorta and the pulmonary artery during ventricular relaxation.

The atrioventricular valves are attached to rings which form the two orifices between atria and ventricles. These rings are made of dense fibrous tissue (*annulus fibrosus*), and the valves themselves are moderately thick, curtain-like structures. The right-sided atrioventricular valve, the *tricuspid valve* (fig. 7), has three leaflets; the left-sided valve, the *mitral valve*, two leaflets. Free edges of each leaflet are connected through a series of delicate strings or cords (*chordae tendineae*) with muscular outgrowths, pillar-like structures, in the lower part of the ventricular cavity (*papillary muscles*). Each ventricle has two such papillary muscles, each connected through the chordae tendineae with free

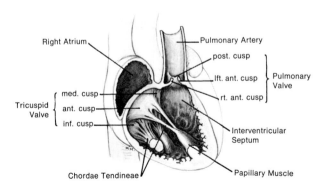

FIGURE 7. *Details of the tricuspid and pulmonary valves.*

edges of the valve leaflets on the respective side. These chordae fan out in a parachute-like fashion to the edge of the valve curtains. The papillary muscle and chordae tendineae stabilize the valves and prevent their flapping back into the atrium in response to the high pressure in the ventricle which closes the valves.

The semilunar valves derive their name from their crescent-shaped leaflets. Each valve consists of three delicate leaflets which are forced apart by high pressure during the ejection of blood into the aorta and the pulmonary artery. These leaflets, or cusps, stay close to the wall of the two arterial trunks, permitting free flow of blood. During the beginning of ventricular relaxation the cusps are sucked back with the blood and completely close the orifice separating the vessels from the ventricles during that portion of the heart cycle.

STRUCTURE OF THE BLOOD VESSELS

The *greater circulation* consists of the aorta, the arteries, the arterioles, the capillary network, and the veins. The aorta and its main tributaries are depicted in figure 8. It is seen that the aorta, after arising from the left ventricle, sends off two coronary arteries, and then runs upward (as the *ascending aorta*), arches to the left (*aortic arch*), and then turns downward, in front of the spinal column, until it reaches the lower abdomen, where it divides into two principal branches. (The more important branches of the aorta are shown in the drawing.) The coronary arteries supply the heart itself; the aorta supplies blood to the head and upper extremities by means of four major arteries: two carotid and two subclavian arteries. On the right side the carotid and subclavian originate as a joint, short trunk (*innominate artery*); on the left side they come off directly from the aorta. The aorta sends off no major branches until it passes below the diaphragm, where three major arteries originate from its frontal wall, and two from its side wall, supplying all abdominal organs. The branches of the coeliac artery supply the stomach, liver, spleen, and pancreas.

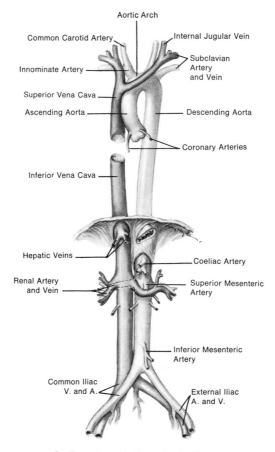

FIGURE 8. *Drawing of the principal arteries and veins. The heart has been removed from the illustration. Only initial portions of smaller vessels are shown. (Abbreviations: a, artery; v, vein.)*

The renal artery supplies the kidneys, and the iliac carries blood to the lower trunk and the legs. The mesenteric artery supplies the intestines.

The *coronary arteries* provide the blood supply for the heart itself (fig. 9). The *left coronary artery* runs a very short course and then divides into two large branches, the *anterior descending coronary artery* and the *left circumflex branch*. The former supplies the front portion of the heart, particularly the left ventricle. The latter branch supplies the lower left portion, the back of the left ventricle, and the left atrium. The *right coronary artery* runs a moderately long course before dividing into branches; it supplies the right side of the heart and the lower back portion of the left ventricle. Even though only two arteries originate from the aorta, the two branches of the left coronary artery are counted as major vessels; thus the clinician is used to thinking in terms of three, rather than two, sources of arterial blood supply to the heart.

The arteries in the body divide and subdivide into smaller segments, similar to branches of a tree. The smallest arterial branches, at the borderline of visibility, are called *arterioles,* beyond which the blood enters myriads of microscopic channels with very thin walls, the *capillaries.* These capillary blood vessels are located within the tissues and organs of the body; they are integral parts of the various organ structures. The capillaries join together into very small veins, *venules,* which in turn join together into increasingly larger veins, eventually forming the two major veins, the superior and inferior vena cava. Larger veins usually accompany corresponding arteries and carry the same names, as indicated in figure 8. The inferior vena cava, the principal lower vein, is

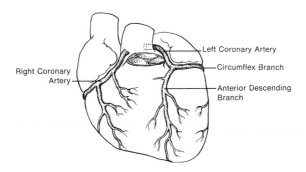

FIGURE 9. *Drawing of the coronary arteries. Description in text.*

located alongside the aorta, deriving tributary veins largely similar to branches of the aorta. It drains blood from the abdomen and the lower part of the body into the right atrium. The large upper vein, the superior vena cava, drains blood from the head and upper extremities through four tributary veins analogous to the four corresponding arterial branches. It runs a short course in the chest, entering the upper portion of the right atrium.

The pulmonary circulation is presented in figure 10. Venous (dark) blood collected in the right atrium is pumped by the right ventricle into the pulmonary artery, which, after a short course upward, divides into two principal branches, each supplying one lung. The right and left branches of the pulmonary artery are large vessels, which are frequently referred to as the "right pulmonary artery" and "left pulmonary artery," in which case the pulmonary artery is called the "pulmonary trunk." Each artery

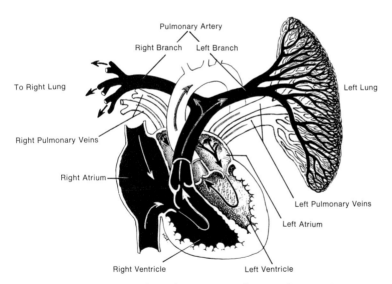

FIGURE 10. *Drawing of the pulmonary circulation. The right lung has been removed from the picture. Sections of the circulation filled with deoxygenated (venous) blood are shown in black; those filled with oxygenated blood in white.*

divides into as many branches as there are lobes of the lungs (three on the right side and two on the left). These branches subdivide further into smaller and smaller branches, forming pulmonary arterioles and then pulmonary capillaries. Capillaries in the lungs have very thin walls separating the blood in them from the air in the *alveoli* (air sacs) of the lungs. Exchange of gases occurs very rapidly and efficiently. The capillaries collect into venules and veins, through which fully oxygenated blood returns to the left side of the heart. The large veins carrying the blood from the lungs to the left atrium number four, two from each lung.

The blood vessels show important structural differences, related to their varying functions. The aorta and the largest of the arteries are thick-walled and quite elastic; smaller arteries have less elastic tissue and more muscular tissue, enabling them to contract and relax. The arterioles have particularly well-developed musculature; their contraction and relaxation is the principal factor in regulating blood pressure, as will be discussed later (chap. 3). The pulmonary artery is thinner than the aorta, as it is exposed to considerably lower pressure. Smaller pulmonary arteries and arterioles have poorly developed musculature, although, in certain diseases, this muscular tissue develops. The veins of the systemic and the pulmonary circuits are thin-walled, collapsible vessels in which blood flows under low pressure. Larger systemic veins have valves (similar to the semilunar valves of the heart) which prevent backflow of blood, particularly in parts of the body where blood flows against the forces of gravity.

The *lymphatic system* is an auxiliary system of blood vessels carrying a white tissue fluid, the *lymph,* resembling blood plasma, which participates in the nutritional process of organs. Most tissues of the body contain lymphatic capillaries, which collect certain elements of tissue fluid and carry it through a fine network into larger vessels and then into a large duct (thoracic duct) which runs upward along the thoracic spine and empties itself into a tributary of the superior vena cava. The lymph thus mixes with blood and becomes part of the blood plasma. Smaller lymphatic vessels are connected with lymph nodes, which act as important filters, extracting undesirable components of tissue fluid and preventing them from entering the bloodstream.

3

The Normal Heart and Circulation: Function

The complicated function of the heart and circulatory system is performed efficiently, with near-perfect coordination. The origin of the heart action lies in a tiny group of cells, a "node" in the upper portion of the heart which acts as a miniature battery, periodically discharging electric current and then recharging itself. Electric current spreads throughout the heart by means of special conduits, wirelike conducting channels. Electric impulses first activate the atria and cause them to contract, and then spread to the two ventricles, making them contract at the optimal time and in a way most advantageous for expelling blood into the great arterial trunks.

The heart is, in physical terms, a pressure pump. It ejects under pressure a certain quantity of blood into a container—the arterial system. Both the pressure and the amount of ejected blood must be carefully regulated by the demands of the body at any given moment. In addition to its over-all regulation of the pumping action, the circulatory system also has the capability to discriminate between the essential and the unessential; for example, during walking, muscles of the legs are adequately supplied with blood at the expense of less essential areas; after meals the digestive organs receive all the blood supply they need.

The most elaborate regulation occurs during exercise. In terms of fuel consumption, the amount of work performed by a marathon runner may be as much as twenty times his minimum need while he is resting. But remarkable work-saving devices within the circulatory system make his heart work only five times as strenuously as during rest.

CONDUCTION OF IMPULSES THROUGH THE HEART

The heart has the unique property of rhythmicity. In order to maintain life it must contract rhythmically seventy times a minute; furthermore, proper function requires a well-coordinated sequence of contractions of its various parts. Rhythmicity and its coordination are dependent upon the function of specialized cells in the heart known as the *conducting system,* which is shown in figure 11. These cells are grouped together into three types of structures: (*a*) two large nodes; (*b*) nervelike conduits, or *bundles*; (*c*) terminal portions of branches of the bundles constituting a fine network at the inner surface of the ventricles. The upper node, the sinoatrial node (*S-A node*), is located at the junction of the superior vena cava and the right atrium. The lower node, the atrioventricular node (*A-V node*), is located in

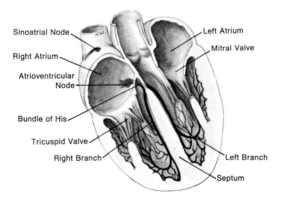

Sinoatrial Node

Right Atrium

Atrioventricular Node

Bundle of His

Tricuspid Valve

Right Branch

Left Atrium

Mitral Valve

Left Branch

Septum

FIGURE 11. *Semidiagrammatic presentation of the heart with its front wall removed, shown to indicate the principal parts of the conducting system. Description in text.*

the lower, septal wall of the right atrium. From the lower portion of the A-V node emerges the *bundle of His,* entering the junction between the two atria and the two ventricles, where it divides into two principal branches, the left bundle branch and the right bundle branch, which run down either side of the ventricular septum. These branches subdivide further into smaller and smaller branches, as shown, and finally connect with the fine network (too small to be drawn) which is located in the endocardial layer of the ventricles, where the conducting system terminates (the *Purkinje network*).

The heart muscle, like other muscular tissue, has the property of contractility—reduction of its length—exerting thereby a considerable force. Since the heart muscle is of globular shape, enveloping a cavity filled with blood, its contraction expels the content of the cardiac cavity. As stated, proper function of the heart as a pump requires coordination of contraction of its muscular structure. This is accomplished by impulses traveling down the conducting system and stimulating muscular tissue to such a contraction. The normal impulse originates in the S-A node, which is usually referred to as the *primary pacemaker.* A strong electrical impulse originates in the S-A nodes; it discharges the impulse and then recharges itself for the next impulse; this occurs on the average of 70 times a minute. The impulse from the S-A node directly stimulates the atria and causes them to contract. At the same time, the impulse is conducted along the inner layer of the atrial musculature, by way of recently identified fibers, to the A-V node. The fast-traveling impulse undergoes considerable slowing when traversing the A-V node from its upper to lower end, but then is rapidly conducted along the bundle of His and its branches to the Purkinje network of each ventricle, producing the well-coordinated contraction of the musculature of the ventricles. The normal duration of the conduction from the atria to the ventricle is just under 0.2 second, so that atrial contraction precedes ventricular contraction by that time interval.

The conducting system has significant built-in safeguards

against failure of the primary pacemaker; each portion of the conducting system has its own property of formation of rhythmical impulse, only weaker and slower than the primary pacemaker. The A-V node constitutes the first line of defense; it comes into operation when signals from the S-A node are not forthcoming and hence it is referred to as the *secondary pacemaker* or *secondary center*. The A-V node discharges usually at a rate of 50 times a minute. The lower parts of the conducting system, that is the bundle of His, its branches, and the Purkinje network, have the weakest and slowest impulse-producing properties; the rate of impulse formation varies from 30 to 50 times per minute. As a rule, the farther away from the A-V node, the slower the rate. Together these lower parts represent the *tertiary pacemaker* or *center,* which only comes into operation in dire emergency when the pathway between the A-V node and the ventricles is interrupted.

The S-A node is connected with the central nervous system through the *autonomic* nervous system. The nervous connections can alter the speed of the impulse formation; the heart rate (originating in the S-A node) speeds up during exercise and excitement and slows down during sleep. The secondary pacemaker has poorer and less efficient nervous regulation of its activity. The tertiary pacemaker has no significant nervous connection, and its rate of discharge is the same under all conditions.

EJECTION OF BLOOD

The pumping action of the heart occurs primarily as a result of ventricular contraction. The atria act more as collecting reservoirs, and their contraction accounts for only a small part of the blood entering the ventricles from the atria; most of it "sucked in" by the ventricles. Since the state of contraction or relaxation of the ventricles determines the over-all volume of the heart, it is customary to divide the cardiac cycle into two periods: the period of ventricular contraction—*systole*; and the period of ventricular relaxation—*diastole.*

During systole, the beginning of ventricular contraction and the resulting first rise in the pressure inside the two ventricular chambers causes the two atrioventricular valves to close (fig. 12a). The sudden tensing of the atrioventicular valves produces a loud sound—the first heart sound. Now the pressure can effectively rise without moving blood from the ventricles until it exceeds the pressure in the aorta and the pulmonary artery, at which point the two semilunar valves are forced open and the flow of blood into the two arterial trunks begins (fig. 12b). Blood is pumped with considerable force and velocity during the first half of the ejection, and then gradually slows down. At the moment of the termination of ventricular contraction and the onset of the period of relaxation (diastole), pressure in the cavities begins to fall, causing immediate closure of semilunar valves, which are "sucked in" into closed position (fig. 12c). Closure of the semilunar valves produces the second heart sound. Relaxation of the ventricular muscle now produces rapid fall in pressure in the two ventricular cavities, and the moment pressure falls below atrial pressures the two atrioventricular valves open widely, permitting the ventricle to fill with blood from the atria (fig. 12d). As stated, relaxation enlarges the ventricular cavities and sucks in atrial blood; this occurs mostly during the earliest one-third of the diastole; during the middle third of that period relatively little pressure change and flow occur. This is the period of "rest," *diastasis*. The final third of diastole involves the contraction of the atria, at which time the small remainder of blood enters the ventricle from the atria (20 percent of the total quantity or less). From the above description, two points are clear. (*a*) During both systole and diastole there are short periods of time during which no flow of blood occurs; these occur between the time one set of valves closes and the other opens, as shown in figures 12a and 12c. These two periods are referred to as *isometric* contraction and relaxation of the cardiac muscle; they are important in permitting rapid rise and fall in pressure to occur efficiently. (*b*) Flow through the two sets of orifices does not occur with uniform volume and velocity; maxi-

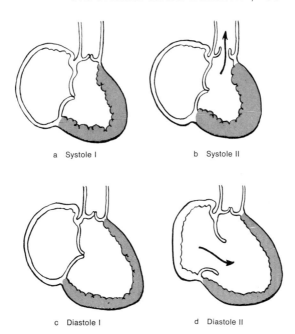

a Systole I   b Systole II

c Diastole I   d Diastole II

FIGURE 12. *Diagrammatic presentation of a ventricle during two stages of systole and two stages of diastole. Description in text.*

mum flow occurs during the earliest part of ventricular ejection and ventricular filling, respectively.

BLOOD PRESSURE AND BLOOD FLOW

During systole the semilunar valves are wide open, and the pressure within the cavities of the two ventricles and the arterial trunks on the respective sides is identical. The highest level of pressure within the ventricle and the arterial system on the corresponding side is called *systolic pressure*. The systolic pressure within the left ventricle and the aorta is about five times higher than the corresponding pressure within the right ventricle and the pulmonary artery. The onset of diastole and closure of semilunar valves signal the separation of pressure between the ventricles and the arterial trunks; pressures in the ventricular cavities drop sharply to levels close to zero; pressures in the aorta and pulmonary artery level off to a point slightly lower than that of semilunar valve closure. The lowest pressure in the ventricles and the lowest pressure levels in the arterial trunks are termed *diastolic pressure*. Since, during most of diastole, pressure in the two ventricles and their respective atria are identical, ventricular diastolic pressure and atrial pressure are usually the same. Normal average pressures in the adult man are as follows:

1) Systolic pressure in the arterial side of the systemic circulation (identical with systolic pressure in the left ventricle): 120 mm. Hg.

2) Diastolic pressure in the aorta and the systemic arteries: 80 mm. Hg.

3) Systolic pressure in the arterial side of the pulmonary circulation and in the right ventricle: 25 mm. Hg.

4) Diastolic pressure in the pulmonary artery and branches: 10 mm. Hg.

5) Pressure in the pulmonary venous side of the circulation, the left atrium, and the left ventricle during diastole: 8 mm. Hg.

6) Pressure in the systemic veins, the right atrium, and the right ventricle during diastole: 3 mm. Hg.

The heart, being a pressure pump, functions properly if it can maintain an adequate flow of blood and adequate pressure. Both blood flow and blood pressure have to be regulated in response to needs of the body. The quantity of blood ejected into each circulatory system—the volume of blood flow—is termed *cardiac output*. Cardiac output can be expressed in two ways: either as the quantity of blood ejected into the arterial system with each ventricular contraction, *stroke volume,* expressed in cubic centimeters per heartbeat; or the total quantity of blood ejected into each arterial system within a minute, *minute volume,* expressed in liters per minute. It is customary to use the general term *cardiac output* to indicate minute volume and to specify stroke volume as such. The maintenance and regulation of cardiac output is one of the most intricate functions of the circulatory system; it will be discussed in connection with the physiology of exercise.

Blood pressure in common usage refers to pressures in the systemic arterial circulation. The level of arterial blood pressure can be maintained at its level of 100 mm. Hg or above only because the blood is enclosed within a system of blood vessels which is so regulated that the same amount of blood which is pumped into it is discharged from it simultaneously. Thus it has to be assumed that if the stroke volume of 70 cc. of blood is ejected into the aorta with each beat, an equal amount leaves the arterial system through the "exit"—the arterioles—into the capillary system. Thus the arterial system is protected at the one end by the aortic valves and at the other end by the sum total of all the arterioles. A simplified diagram of such a system is drawn in figure 13, in which a pump (at left) is shown to eject fluid into an elastic container which has at its end a stopcock and which is connected to a much larger container from which a system of tubes returns the fluid into the pump. The pump can be imagined to imitate the left side of the heart; the first "closed" container the high-pressure arterial system; the "stopcock" represents the arterioles; the larger, open container represents the capillary and venous reservoir of blood; the returning pipes the larger veins; and the lower left container the atria. The arterioles

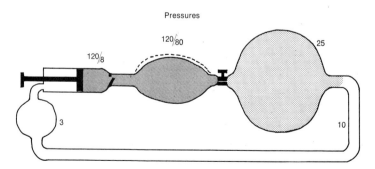

FIGURE 13. *Drawing of a circulatory model resembling the human circulation. Description in text.*

are normally in a semiconstricted state and are regulated by impulses reaching them from the central nervous system via the nerves. These impulses are capable of either constricting further or relaxing the arterioles, thereby regulating outflow from the first reservoir, and through this the arterial pressure. The arterioles taken together represent the resistance to blood flow as a stopcock in physics experiments is used to regulate pressure. In the arterial system this resistance is very high; in the pulmonary arterial system arterioles are wide open, and hence resistance and pressures are much lower than on the systemic side. The capillary and venous systems in both circuits have no narrow area offering any resistance to flow, and hence their pressure is close to zero. This relationship between pressure, flow, and resistance is usually presented in the form of an equation, which is a derivative of Poiseuille's law and is analogous to Ohm's law in electricity:

Pressure equals *flow* (cardiac output) times *resistance:*
$$P = F \times R$$

It follows that pressure can be maintained at a constant level only if resistance falls each time cardiac output increases. This actually takes place because of a well-regulated barostat, a mechanism analogous to the thermostat which is widely used to maintain temperature at a constant level in homes or appliances. The thermostat represents a heat-sensitive detector which shuts off heat production when temperature rises, and increases it with falling temperature. The human barostat consists of pressure-sensitive points within the walls of some arteries. If the ejection of the blood into the aorta increases, raising the cardiac output, the aorta is filled with more blood and is more distended. Pressure-sensitive receptors sense the distension of arterial walls and send appropriate signals through the nervous system which lead to relaxation of arterioles just the proper amount to let the excess blood out of the arterial system and to maintain arterial pressure at the previous level.

The systemic circulation consists of many circuits connected in parallel (see fig. 1). Each of these smaller circuits has its own resistance at the arteriolar level. The general equation mentioned above applies to each of these circuits as well as to their sum total; consequently, arteriolar resistance in each region determines its flow independently within the over-all flow and pressure available. Thus, if in a given organ the arterioles were to constrict, its blood supply would be reduced, since blood would more easily go through alternate circuits; if arteriolar relaxation occurred in a given circuit, *more* blood would flow through it than the proportional share of the total. This mechanism, mediated less through the central nervous system and more through local reflexes, controls blood flow through individual organs and parts of the body. Such a regulating mechanism (*regional flow control*) is of considerable importance in the efficient functioning of our body. It provides for an increased blood flow in areas where it is most needed; thus, during exercise the working muscles receive a more abundant blood supply. After meals the digestive tract is provided with increased blood flow, and this may occur without disrupting the general balance of the total flow or altering the arterial pressure in the systemic circulation.

The blood pressure is the same in all arteries up to the beginning of the arterioles. There the pressure falls abruptly from a systolic level of 120 mm. Hg to a pressure of 25 mm. Hg in the capillaries, which is just sufficient to drive the blood into the venous system through the narrow capillary channels. On the venous side blood flows at low velocity toward the heart. The veins have virtually no driving power, and the blood flow is aided by the venous valves and by the massaging action of the various muscles of the body.

The aorta and its principal branches are, as mentioned, elastic vessels. This property plays an important part in making the blood flow through the body evenly, rather than intermittently. During systole all the elastic arteries are expanded by the addition of blood ejected from the left ventricle; when the ejection of blood is ended the elastic vessels come down to their original size as the excess blood is being eliminated into the capillaries.

If blood were ejected into a system of totally rigid pipes, then forward flow of blood would occur only during the systole and would stop during diastole. Elastic tissue in arterial walls makes for a reservoir of variable capacity which acts as a pressure and flow equalizer. This principle is often used in perfume and cologne spray dispensers: simple dispensers with one bulb spray only when the bulb is squeezed; dispensers with a double bulb are capable of spraying continuously even though the bulb is squeezed intermittently because the second bulb (which is not squeezed) distends with air when the first bulb is squeezed and acts as a pressure and flow equalizer.

The sudden dilation of the aorta by the blood ejected from the left ventricle is transmitted along the arterial system as a wave of elastic displacement of the arterial wall. This represents the arterial pulse wave, usually referred to as the *arterial pulse*. The pulse is an index of the heart rate, but, in addition, reflects the quantity of blood ejected into the aorta, the mode of its injection, the elasticity of the larger arteries, and the condition of the "closed" arterial system. It obviously provides important and readily obtainable information concerning the circulatory apparatus. A study of the arterial pulse has been a basis of diagnosis of disease for many centuries.

The circulation through the pulmonary circuit (*lesser circulation*) is very much simpler than the systemic circulation. It is confined to within a single organ, the lungs; therefore there is little need for the regulation of blood flow (see fig. 4). Its pressure is low under normal circumstances (see above), because pulmonary arterioles are wide open and offer little resistance to flow, and, under ordinary circumstances, nervous regulation of pulmonary arterioles is practically nonexistent. Consequently the fall in pressure from the arteriolar side to the capillary side of the pulmonary circulation (*gradient of pressure*) is very low, less than 10 mm. Hg.

It has been stated in the previous chapter that the final destination of the circulatory system is the capillary network of both circuits. In it all the exchanges between blood and tissue, and between blood and air, take place. The thinness of the capillary walls, permitting easy exchanges of material through it, has already been stressed. These walls act as semipermeable membranes through which water and chemical substances dissolved in the blood plasma can enter and exit as needed, driven by two forces: the osmotic pressure on the two sides of the capillary walls and the hydrostatic pressure within them. Each substance dissolved in the blood on one side of the capillary wall, and in the tissue fluid on its other side, reaches an equilibrium in the two media. The pressure in the capillaries is measured at about 25 mm. Hg which maintains a fluid balance within the vascular system, as this pressure is identical with the osmotic pressure exerted by plasma proteins and electrolytes. If the hydrostatic pressure increases, or the osmotic pressure falls, then fluid tends to leave the vascular system, increasing the fluid content of tissues—a situation which then may lead to edema (to be discussed in chap. 5). Fall in hydrostatic pressure or increase in osmotic pressure draws fluid into the vascular system, increasing the circulating blood volume. These factors play an important role in the mechanism maintaining the volume of blood at an optimal level. Water and solutes undergo exchange in the capillary system with great speed and efficiency. Exchange of blood gases—oxygen and carbon dioxide—takes place across the capillary wall with even greater speed and efficiency. The objectives of these gas exchanges have already been discussed.

EXERCISE

The circulatory system provides a means of supplying oxygen and other vital substances to tissues of the body. Obviously, the demands upon this supply line increase sharply during performance of exercise. Human energy is customarily expressed in terms of utilization of oxygen from air (*oxygen consumption*); oxygen consumption is to the body what gasoline consumption is to the automobile. The oxygen consumption reaches its minimum during complete rest (*resting oxygen consumption*) and measures in an average adult between 200 and 250 cc. of oxygen per minute. This covers the basal metabolic needs of the body (*basal metabolism*). The level of oxygen consumption increases very steeply with activity, since the oxygen cost of human effort is quite high. For example, walking at a moderate pace increases oxygen consumption about three times its basal level. Strenuous exercise, such as climbing stairs briskly, or running, may increase the basal demands for oxygen by as much as five to eight times. Maximum possible effort for a healthy individual occurs at the cost of 10 to 15 times the basal oxygen consumption; for a trained athlete it may reach 20 times the resting level. This high need for oxygen is one of the principal limiting factors of human exercise. The limitation depends upon the possible top performance of the two principal systems involved in the process: (*a*) respiration, supplying enough oxygen to the air spaces of the lungs; and (*b*) circulation, delivering enough oxygen to the working tissues. The burden of delivering 10 to 20 times the basal amount of oxygen to the tissues is very considerable, and is only possible because of work-saving adaptive mechanisms. These adaptive mechanisms apply primarily to the circulatory apparatus, since the respiration is usually capable of increasing its work in proportion to high demands, while the circulatory system is not. On the other hand, the circulatory system is so designed that delivery of oxygen can increase much more than the work of the heart and circulation can. This is made possible through three adaptive mechanisms:

1) The available oxygen supply is more fully utilized. This is made easy by the fact that normally during rest only a small part of the available oxygen is consumed by the tissues. Blood returning to the right side of the heart is, at rest, still 75 percent saturated with oxygen, indicating that only one-fourth of the available supply has been utilized. Better utilization of oxygen provides a very effective work-saving device for the heart. For example, if a certain form of exercise demands *four* times the resting amount, the tissue can easily draw *twice* as much oxygen as during rest (reducing the oxygen saturation of the returning

venous blood from the normal of 75 to 50 percent), in which case the volume of blood circulating through the tissues (cardiac output) has to increase only *twice* instead of four times to meet the full demand.

2) Blood can be redistributed (by way of regional flow regulation, as discussed earlier) in such a manner that the working muscles or organs get a higher share of the total at the expense of reduced flow through less important regions. Thus, during muscular exercise, the digestive tract, the kidneys, the brain, the skin, and other nonparticipating organs are perfused with *less* blood than during rest, in order to supply the heart and the working muscles with more oxygen.

3) Working muscles can perform temporarily with an oxygen supply smaller than the actual energy needs, thereby drawing an "oxygen debt," which is repaid immediately after cessation of exercise. This mechanism is particularly important for short-term, violent forms of exercise.

These adaptive mechanisms are essential, since the heart has rather limited capacity for increase in its work. It is estimated that in a healthy individual cardiac output can only increase to a maximum of four or five times its resting level (from a normal of 5 liters per minute to 20 or 25 liters per minute), the lower figure probably representing the more realistic average value. Thus, as a general rule, one can assume that the heart reaches its ceiling of performance by increasing its work (and potential oxygen supply to the tissues) fourfold; the tissues can extract up to four times as much oxygen from the blood during exercise than at rest; therefore, top muscular performance is about 16 times the resting level when expressed in terms of oxygen consumption.

The following illustration may help the reader comprehend the adaptive circulatory process during exercise: Let us imagine a large industrial plant with diversified activities, which has ample supplies of raw material but has no storage facilities for its principal fuel, coal, which has to be brought in as it is needed. The ordinary, minimal manufacturing activities of the plant are met by a daily quantity of coal, equivalent to five carloads; however, since the shortest train consists of 20 cars, coal is brought in daily in such a train and one-quarter of each car is unloaded, thereby supplying the needs. At times the plant is called upon to increase temporarily the manufacture of one of its principal products. The increased fuel demands are met in part by bringing in longer trains, and in part by unloading a higher fraction of each car. The plant can also, in order to conserve fuel, slow down or eliminate the manufacture of some less essential product. If one assumes that the rail loading facilities at the other end of the communication line limit coal delivery to 80 carloads a day, the maximum manufacturing capabilities of the plant would amount to 16 times its ordinary level, if all 80 carloads were brought in and all the coal in them unloaded.

Physiologists and clinicians often find it necessary to calculate the work of the heart at rest and during exercise. This is usually expressed in terms of work delivered (*external work*) rather than the actual energy utilized by the heart. External work is expressed by the formula:

Work equals *blood pressure* times *cardiac output:*

$$W = P \times F$$

The increase in work during exercise is directly related to the increase in cardiac output, since blood pressure shows little change, its level being well regulated by the previously described barostatic mechanism.

In spite of the very efficient work-saving devices for the heart and the circulation which operate in the healthy individual, exercise imposes heavy strain upon the circulatory system. Obviously, under conditions of less than perfect health, certain functions of the circulation begin to lag and the efficiency of the circulatory adjustment may suffer. Exercise may, therefore, bring forth findings which suggest faulty circulatory function long before it becomes evident under resting conditions. Exercise thus provides one of the fundamental tests of the circulatory apparatus in the study of cardiac disease.

Part Two

The Abnormal Heart: A General Approach

4

Diagnosis

Medical diagnosis represents a process of intricate deduction which somewhat resembles crime detection. It was no coincidence that the most celebrated mystery writer of all times, Sir Arthur Conan Doyle, was a physician. His Sherlock Holmes was patterned after his teacher in medical school in Edinburgh, Dr. Joseph Bell, who was a superb diagnostician and made a profound impression upon the young student by his brilliant deductions from medical clues.

In the diagnosis of diseases of the heart and circulation, the physician obtains his initial clues from the medical history and the physical examination. Afterward, further information may be obtained by the various auxiliary methods of examination and laboratory procedures, which range all the way from simple tests performed in the doctor's office to the most complex procedures available only in major medical centers. The physician is always the central figure in the process of sifting the evidence—the master detective who has to know which clues to follow and who decides at which point his case is completed.

In this chapter the various methods used in the diagnosis of cardiovascular diseases are discussed. The presentation is concerned mainly with the purpose of the diagnostic methods, rather than their substance; it emphasizes the why's, rather than the how's.

CASE FINDING

In the majority of cases the diagnostic evaluation of a patient suspected of having heart disease represents the first contact between the patient and the physician. The average patient consults the physician because of certain symptoms which make him believe that his health may be less than perfect. However, in recent years there has been an ever-growing proportion of patients who see a physician for reasons other than symptoms and their belief that they may be ill. This is the result of a procedure referred to as "case finding."

Case finding is a process which was first initiated by health authorities in tracing the origin of infectious diseases, such as tuberculosis. This process has been widened to include diseases other than communicable ones, in line with the increasing interest in the important field of preventive medicine, devoted to the idea that early discovery of disease may prevent its progression or make a cure easier. In cardiovascular diseases case finding is helped by various mass surveys including X rays, electrocardiograms, and other tests. Some individuals are referred to physicians as a result of pre-employment examinations, insurance examinations, or periodic health examinations. Consequently, a significant proportion of individuals are now examined for possible heart disease as a result of suspicion which has originated in a survey or "routine" health examination. Among abnormalities brought to light during such procedures are the following:

1) A heart murmur, or an irregularity of the heartbeat, discovered during routine "check-up" in children.

2) Heart murmurs, high blood pressure, or irregularity of heart action found in pre-employment examinations, insurance examinations, or periodic health examinations.

3) Enlargement of the heart, or an unusual shape, revealed by chest X rays taken in a mass survey or as part of a routine examination.

4) Suspicious abnormalities suggestive of heart disease as

shown by electrocardiograms, taken during a "routine physical."

The importance of such findings to the individual in whom they are detected varies considerably. In many such cases, significant heart disease has later been ruled out altogether; in others, heart disease may be confirmed but found to be inconsequential to the general health of the individual. There is, however, a significant yield of cases of important heart disease discovered in this manner in individuals who considered themselves in good health and who would otherwise not have sought medical care. Even among those there are instances in which such a discovery may not significantly alter the course of the disease, and the early knowledge of heart disease may not benefit the individual. Yet in some cases, early recognition of heart disease may be of great benefit to the individual, for treatment at that point may lead to control of the disease, or may even permit a complete cure. Early discovery of heart disease is of particular importance to young individuals with organic heart disease in whom vocational guidance may represent an important asset later in life. It is important, however, for the physician to consider the potential harm done to an individual in good health, or one with a trivial heart problem, who becomes "heart conscious" and develops undue anxiety about the condition of his heart as a result of the mere suspicion of heart disease.

Thus, case findings as applied to heart disease has to be considered less important than in either communicable disease or cancer. In the former, the whole community may benefit by the finding of an unknown case of tuberculosis or a similar disease; in the latter case, early discovery of cancer is always of benefit to the individual in whom it is found, and is often responsible for saving his life. However, in the field of cardiovascular disease, case finding may greatly benefit some individuals, be a matter of indifference to others, and may even be deleterious to some by starting them on the road to anxiety and neurosis. Thus, case finding in heart disease requires real understanding and a great deal of wisdom on the part of the physician.

MEDICAL HISTORY

The medical history is usually obtained by the physician during his initial contact with the patient. It consists of a lengthy interview, at which time the physician not only listens to the patient describing his various complaints, if any, but, by means of a skillful cross-examination, also tries to assess the patient's personality, reliability, power of observation, memory, and his attitude toward disease. The physician usually tries to interpret the patient's symptoms in the light of his motivation. The average patient consults the physician out of a genuine concern about his health; however, there are situations in which the patient could benefit either by concealing his symptoms or by overstating them. The former situation may arise in the course of a pre-employment or insurance examination; the latter problem concerns health claims and disability benefits. The experienced physician can usually form a reasonable picture of the patient's symptoms undistorted by bias provided he deals with a person of some reliability and intelligence.

The contribution of the medical history to the diagnosis of heart disease shows a very wide range. In some cases the history contributes nothing to the diagnosis; in others, diagnosis may depend altogether upon the history. Between these extremes lies an entire spectrum, but it is fair to say that, on the average, the medical history plays a very significant role in the over-all diagnostic evaluation of a patient with heart disease, particularly on the crucial point of whether there is disability, and its extent and progression.

In strict medical terminology, disease presents itself by symptoms (subjective manifestations) and signs (objective manifestations). This distinction is sometimes obliterated by the common usage of the two terms, in which they overlap or are used interchangeably. In heart disease there are two principal subjective manifestations which could be termed "cardinal" symptoms: *dyspnea* (shortness of breath) and *chest pain*.

Shortness of breath is a symptom which is not only important but also exceedingly difficult to analyze and evaluate. There are several reasons for this. In the first place, dyspnea is not a new or unaccustomed sensation to an individual: everyone, when running or climbing stairs rapidly becomes short of breath; consequently, dyspnea, as a manifestation of disease, merely represents the patient's impression that certain activity evokes shortness of breath to a greater extent than he had expected. Unless shortness of breath occurs at rest or with only minor activity, the estimation on the part of the patient may be unreliable. Furthermore, shortness of breath is not a specific symptom of heart disease; it occurs in many forms of diseases of the lungs, the chest, in anemia, in some forms of cancer, and other conditions. Finally, the essence of dyspnea is hard to define, for the physician may observe a patient having obviously labored respiration and yet have him deny "shortness of breath," while another individual claims to experience dyspnea at a time when his respiration appears perfectly normal. The most widely accepted definition of dyspnea is "consciousness of an increased effort of respiration." Dyspnea is related to the need for additional oxygen for the performance of exercise. As explained in chapter 3, the respiratory apparatus has to supply the needed oxygen by providing deeper and faster breathing. This occurs automatically, without the individual's at first being conscious of the increased respiratory effort, but when his capability reaches the peak he experiences the sensation of shortness of breath. In patients with heart disease the lungs are stiffer, and the "ceiling" of respiratory effort associated with the sensation of dyspnea occurs with much less effort.

Shortness of breath associated with less exercise than the individual is used to performing easily is the commonest form of dyspnea of heart disease and is termed *effort dyspnea*. It represents one of the most frequent limiting factors for exercise; it therefore produces disability. The physician recording the patient's history usually interprets dyspnea in the light of the patient's customary activities: a trained athlete with heart disease may have significant effort dyspnea but still be able to perform everyday activities; a sedentary worker may be hardly aware of increasing cardiac disability due to dyspnea simply because he does not perform enough exercise to become aware of it.

Abnormal shortness of breath may also occur when the patient is resting. This occurs most commonly at night, particularly during sleep: the patient is awakened with a feeling of intense air hunger and suffocation. This form of dyspnea is referred to as *paroxysmal nocturnal dyspnea*. Milder forms of it often subside spontaneously; the patient usually gets out of bed, sits up, or walks to the open window: after a few moments the attack subsides. In its more severe form such dyspnea may be associated with expectoration of pink and frothy sputum; it is then termed *acute pulmonary edema,* a particularly dangerous form of dyspnea. Sometimes dyspnea of heart disease is associated with coughing and wheezing—*cardiac asthma*. All these forms of shortness of breath at rest which are caused by heart disease are associated with failure of the left ventricle.

The physician taking the patient's history and convincing himself that the patient does indeed have significant shortness of breath then has to gather clues from the history to decide whether the dyspnea is due to heart disease, to diseases of the lungs, or to other causes. Sometimes information obtained from the history permits the identification of the underlying disease; in other cases, the decision has to await examination and special tests.

The other cardinal symptom of cardiac disease is pain. In contrast to dyspnea, chest pain is not an accentuated normal reaction but is always abnormal. However, chest pain is not always a manifestation of heart disease, or even of serious disease at all. To be sure, chest pain may indicate serious heart disease, diseases of the lungs, chest wall, spine, and many other structures; yet it is commonly a trivial manifestation of muscle ache or strained muscles or ligaments which produces undue anxiety in an individual who may associate it with heart disease. The identification of the nature of chest pain and its possible relationship to heart disease is a difficult task for the physician, and is a real challenge; it often requires a good deal of experience, patience, and ingenuity.

Chest pain due to cardiac disease, *cardiac pain,* is related to inadequate blood flow through the heart, thereby representing a symptom of coronary disease. It is assumed that the painful sensation is due to signals originating in the heart when a certain portion of the heart muscle is temporarily deprived of oxygen, in which case its metabolism produces some abnormal substances (lactic acid or the like) which send pain signals. In milder cases of coronary artery disease, lack of oxygen to the heart muscle (*ischemia*) occurs only during increased work load, such as exercise or excitement. In more advanced cases pain may occur at rest.

In addition to the two cardinal symptoms of heart disease discussed in detail, there are many other symptoms about which the physician inquires when taking the history, or which are reported to him by the patient. Among these are: "palpitations," various sensations related to the patient's consciousness of unusual heart action, mostly related to irregularities of heartbeat; dizziness; faintness or attacks of fainting; undue tiredness; headaches; abdominal pain; and many others. Furthermore, the physician obtains information from the patient concerning *his* observation of certain signs (objective manifestations of disease) such as swelling of legs, unexplained changes in body weight, abnormal color (jaundice, blueness of parts of the body), and so forth.

In the search for important clues in the diagnosis of heart disease it is necessary to review certain points from the patient's past: information thus obtained may help clarify the nature of heart disease. Among the more significant clues in the past history are the following: (*a*) history of rheumatic fever in childhood; (*b*) information concerning the discovery of heart disease in early infancy, thereby suggesting its congenital origin; (*c*) history of infectious diseases—diphtheria, tuberculosis, endocarditis, syphilis; (*d*) the patient's dietary, tobacco, and alcohol habits; (*e*) family background concerning such traits as coronary disease, hypertension, and diabetes; (*f*) glandular disorders; and many others.

The medical history usually gives the physician enough information to evaluate the problem in a preliminary way; he can then proceed to the next step, the physical examination, with certain specific ideas of the problem at hand.

PHYSICAL EXAMINATION

It is axiomatic that each patient suspected of having heart disease has to undergo a complete physical examination. Certain parts of the physical examination are of particular significance in the diagnosis of cardiovascular disease, and these will be discussed briefly. Among there are: (*a*) examination of the heart itself; (*b*) examination of the peripheral circulation; (*c*) examination of those other organs which are often affected by improper performance of the heart.

The traditional examination of the heart consists of inspection, percussion, palpation, and auscultation of the region of the chest overlying the heart. Of these, percussion is the least reliable method and has been abandoned altogether in some clinics. Inspection and palpation of the chest, together, do provide significant information in heart disease, as they may uncover abnormal motion due to overactivity of heart action, hypertrophy of either of the two ventricles, abnormal areas of pulsation, and "palpable" (unusually forceful and loud) heart sounds and murmurs.

The auscultation of the heart is the key to physical examination in heart disease. In recent years, thanks to newer physiological studies of the circulation and their correlation with examination of the heart, auscultation has become a more scientific method of examination. The subjects of auscultation are: (*a*) heart sounds; (*b*) heart murmurs; and (*c*) "added" sound phenomena.

The normal heart produces two loud noises, called *heart sounds*. These sounds coincide with closure of the two sets of valves (see chap. 2), and therefore signify the onset of systole or diastole, respectively. The "first" heart sound is caused by tensing and closure of the mitral and tricuspid valves and occurs with the beginning of ventricular contraction; the "second" heart sound is caused by closure of the two semilunar valves, signifying the beginning of diastole. In addition to the first and second heart sounds, there are two more sounds which are seldom heard in health but are often present in heart disease. These are the third heart sound, coincidental with rapid filling of the ventricles, often referred to as the *ventricular gallop sound*; and the fourth heart sound related to atrial contraction (*atrial gallop sound*). The diagnostic value of heart sounds is considerable. Alteration of the two "normal" heart sounds, such as increase or decrease in their intensity and their splitting into two components, may provide information concerning the state of the valves, pressure changes within the heart, or a relationship between the dynamic events within the two ventricles. The prominent appearance of the "gallop" sounds occurs in heart failure and in the presence of unusual rapidity of blood flow through the heart due to a variety of causes.

Heart murmurs are produced by vibrations and acoustical fluctuation when blood flowing at high velocity meets an obstacle, such as an abrupt narrowing of its channel. Such circumstances occur under the following conditions:

1) Narrowing of any of the four valvular orifices of the heart;

2) Incomplete closure of a valve, permitting regurgitation of blood in an abnormal direction;

3) An opening between the two ventricles (usually a birth defect);

4) Communication between the arterial system and a low-pressure system (such as the pulmonary circulation or the venous system);

5) Areas of localized narrowing within the arterial system.

In addition, certain vibrations, similar to heart murmurs, may originate outside the heart but be mistaken for heart murmurs.

Murmurs play an important role in the diagnosis of heart disease. In some cases the heart murmur alone may permit a positive identification of a specific form of heart disease; in other cases it may represent the basis for further search by various tests. However, heart murmurs appear frequently without significant heart disease and even occur in entirely healthy individuals; consequently proper evaluation of cardiac murmurs requires a good deal of thought and experience.

Added sound phenomena may provide useful diagnostic information. For example, a sound in early diastole is often associated with the opening of the mitral valve if it is thickened and diseased (*mitral opening snap*). Blood ejected into a dilated aorta or pulmonary artery produces an additional sound in systole (*ejection click*); diseases of the pericardium may be associated with added sounds or with a characteristic noise, caused by the heart rubbing against roughened pericardium, which resembles squeaking leather (*pericardial friction rub*).

Physical examination of the heart is a difficult and yet a rewarding part of the diagnostic evaluation of the patient. Its finesses can only be appreciated after considerable training and experience; astute cardiologists can often derive amazingly accurate information about the circulatory system without added laboratory procedures. Yet there are certain problems which present difficulties even to experts. One of the most perplexing of these is the separation of an "innocent" heart murmur from a murmur indicative of disease. In the present era of available surgical treatment of certain forms of heart disease, such diagnostic problems often have to be carried to ultimate tests, such as cardiac catheterization, in order to resolve it beyond a reasonable doubt.

Physical examination of the vascular system involves:

1) Measurement of the blood pressure.
2) Examination of the arterial system.
3) Examination of the venous system.

Arterial blood pressure is determined with the aid of the well-known blood pressure apparatus, the sphygmomanometer, which is available either as a mercury manometer or as a spring manometer (aneroid). Blood pressure is measured by inflating a rubber cuff to a pressure higher than that within the artery of an arm or leg, thereby interrupting the blood flow. When the cuff is deflated, the blood will start flowing into the obstructed limb and the onset of blood flow under the cuff will be signified by a sound, which will be heard when the pressure in the cuff (read on the manometer) equals the systolic pressure in the artery underneath. This sound occurs coincidentally with each heartbeat and can be heard by placing a stethoscope over the artery beneath the inflated cuff. When the cuff is further deflated the sound disappears or becomes muffled. This occurs when the pressure in the cuff equals the diastolic pressure in the constricted artery. Ordinarily blood pressure is the same in all the arteries; differences in pressure between the two arms or between arms and legs usually signifies the presence of an obstruction in front of the area of lower pressure.

Examination of the arterial system consists of palpation, or examination by touch, of all arteries that are superficially located. This usually includes arteries in the upper extremities, lower extremities, and neck; in thinner individuals it is possible to palpate the abdominal aorta. Palpation of the arteries permits the examination of the arterial pulse and the estimation of undue thickness and tortuosity of the arterial walls. Absence of pulsation or unequal pulsation between two sides of the body suggests some arterial obstruction. Examination of the pulse provides information beyond that pertaining to the local condition of the given artery. As explained in chapter 3, the pulse gives an insight into the rate and rhythm, the stroke volume, and the state of the arterial tree. Specific abnormalities of the pulse (such as a rapidly rising and "collapsing" pulse, or a slow rising small pulse) often are associated with specific diseases of the heart and circulation. Alternation of stronger and weaker pulse beats is often found in heart failure (*pulsus alternans*); unusual variation of the pulse with respiration may be present in diseases of the pericardium (*pulsus paradoxus*).

While palpation of the arterial pulse indicates the condition of the major arteries and conveys information transmitted from the heart, smaller arterial channels and the peripheral circulation as a whole can be assessed roughly by examination of the parts of the body furthest from the heart: the feet and hands. Two features are of particular importance: the color and temperature of the extremities. While both these features show great individual variation, a difference between the two extremities in an individual strongly suggests some disturbance of the circulation within one of them.

Examination of the venous system consists of inspection and palpation of the major veins and examination of the venous pulse. Inspection of veins, particularly in the extremities, permits the detection of such abnormalities as varicose veins. Palpation of veins may permit the detection of thrombi (clots) in them. Examination of the venous pulse can only be done by inspection, since the low-pressure venous system does not have a pulse strong enough to be palpable. The venous pulse, usually observed in the neck, provides useful information concerning the performance of the right side of the heart, since it directly reflects pulse waves from the right atrium.

Examination of other parts of the body specifically affected in diseases of the heart and circulation may reveal a variety of information: the lungs may make bubbling respiratory noises (rales) signifying congestion due to heart failure; the skin and mucous membranes (such as the lips) may show cyanosis (bluish discoloration caused by lower content of oxygen in the blood flowing through them); inspection of the skin and the membranes of the eye may disclose jaundice; the liver and spleen, which can be palpated when examining the abdomen, may be found to be enlarged, or there may be edema (swelling of the subcutaneous tissue, usually most noticeable around the ankles). Many other organs or bodily areas, such as the thyroid gland, the joints, the fingertips, and the nail beds, when diseased, may provide background information about the type of heart disease.

After completing the history and physical examination the physician can usually arrive at a tentative diagnosis. Such a diagnosis may be firm and accurate in some cases, awaiting only confirmation by further tests; in other cases the information obtained may be contradictory and confusing, and further diagnostic procedures may appear essential. In any case, the physician has reached the point where he has to decide which further procedures are needed. It has already been stated that diagnostic procedures fall into two categories: those readily available to all physicians, and those of complex nature which are performed in a "cardiac laboratory." The key procedures in the former category are:

X ray examination of the heart (radiologic examination) and electrocardiographic examination.

RADIOLOGIC EXAMINATION

The X ray examination of the heart provides the most reliable method for the assessment of the size and shape of the heart. Such an examination usually consists of the observation of the heart shadow on the radiolucent screen (fluoroscopy) and the recording of the heart shadow on film with a tube-target distance of six feet. The latter method is the more important one, as it provides a permanent record which can be studied in detail and which may serve as the basis for future comparison. The standard chest X ray is usually taken on a 14 by 17 inch film. The examination generally includes four such films taken at different degrees of rotation.

The principle of X ray examination of the heart is based on the fact that the chest consists of two media: the lungs, which, by virtue of their high content of air, are highly radiolucent (transparent to X rays); and the heart and great vessels, which are radioopaque, and therefore cast a shadow in relation to the lungs upon the screen or film. Bones are even more radioopaque than the heart, and calcium within the cardiovascular system can be identified by a deeper density than the remainder of the shadow. The size and shape of the heart shadow in the varying degrees of rotation provides not only information concerning over-all cardiac enlargement but also the recognition of which of the four cardiac chambers are enlarged. The great vessels, the aorta and pulmonary artery and their branches, can be identified and deviations in their size and shape can be recognized. Finally, the circulation through the lung is easily visible; the number and size of small vessels in the lungs may indicate increased or decreased blood flow to the lungs or congestion of the lungs. As mentioned, calcium deposits are readily visible; examination of the various views may help in identifying their presence in the heart valves, the aorta. the coronary arteries, or the pericardium.

The four standard positions in which films are taken are termed:

(*a*) anteroposterior (front to back; see fig. 14); (*b*) lateral (side to side); (*c*) right anterior oblique (right shoulder forward); and (*d*) left anterior oblique (left shoulder forward). The last two views are taken at roughly 45 degrees to the first two. It is also customary to give the patient a tablespoon of barium paste to swallow, which opacifies the esophagus. The esophagus is located directly behind the heart and is displaced backwards when the heart enlarges. Opacification of the esophagus is particularly important for the detection of enlargement of the left atrium.

In addition to the standard radiologic methods mentioned above, there are special techniques sometimes applicable for the study of the heart and great vessels. Among these are roentgen-kymography, a study of the motion of the border of the heart shadow taken with a series of slits; and tomography, a series of films taken with the X-ray tubes rotating around the object, which explores specific depths of the heart shadow. These methods are used less frequently than in the past; newer and more precise methods have largely replaced them in cases where more detail is needed than the standard film can supply. These special tech-

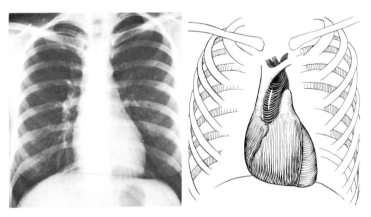

FIGURE 14. *An X-ray film of the chest in the anteroposterior view in a healthy individual. The reference diagram at the right shows the heart and the great vessels in relation to the rib cage. Compare with figure 5 to identify cardiovascular structures.*

niques will be discussed in connection with the cardiac laboratory.

The contribution of standard radiography to the diagnosis of diseases of the heart and circulation is a major one. Enlargement of the heart is one of the most important signs of heart disease; changes of heart size occurring in serial film provide valuable information concerning progress of disease or response to treatment; the analysis of heart chamber sizes aids in the diagnosis of specific diseases; important diagnostic conclusions can be obtained from abnormalities noted in the great vessels and the lung fields. Of all the laboratory methods supplementing the physical examination, radiography is probably the most important.

ELECTROCARDIOGRAPHY

Electrocardiography is the other widely used essential method of heart study. This technique is universally available and has become part of the "routine" examination of the heart. The electrocardiograph is an apparatus which records highly amplified electrical impulses originating with each heartbeat. Its proper role in the diagnosis can best be comprehended if its theoretical basis is briefly explained.

It has been mentioned in chapter 3 that the heart muscle consists of two types of cells: the contracting muscle fibers and the special cells of the conducting system. Each cell of either kind can be considered a miniature battery, which discharges electricity (electrical potential) while active and which recharges itself during the period of rest. The process of discharge of electrical potential is called *depolarization,* and the recharging, *repolarization.* The discharge of electricity from each cell is measurable and can be recorded by appropriately sensitive galvanometers. The electrocardiograph is such a galvanometer adapted for the amplification and recording of the stronger signals from the heart. It is obvious that it would be impracticable to record and measure electric potential at its source—the heart cells. In order to utilize this method in humans the electrical potential has to be recorded from easily accessible points of the body some distance from the origin of the signals. Thus, electrical signals originating in the heart are filtered through various parts of the body, which act as conductors of electricity; far removed from the source, the electrocardiograph can only record the strongest signals. Under ordinary circumstances there are three strong groups of electrical signals which can be picked up from the body surface:

1) The discharge of potential produced by the activation and depolarization of the atria; this is a relatively weak signal, recorded as a gentle peak.

2) The strong signal produced by depolarization of the ventricles and occurring just before cardiac contraction; this is shown as a sharp multiphasic deflection.

3) The smaller and gentler wave signifying the repolarization (recharging) of the ventricles.

Weaker signals, such as the origin of the impulse in the pacemaker, its transmission through the conducting system, or the recharging of the atria are not detectable by the conventional electrocardiograph. The various complexes are labeled by letters: the depolarization of the atria is called the P-wave; the depolarization of the ventricles, the QRS-complex; and the repolarization of the ventricle, the T-wave. A typical electrocardiographic lead is shown in figure 15. Electric potential represents the movement of electrons; since it is not possible to record the potential of every cell separately, the potential recorded in the electrocardiogram represents the sum total of all electrical discharges, and represents the spread of activation of electricity through the various portions of the heart. The galvanometer records the difference in potential between the two points: in electrocardiography the two points represent a proximal (exploring) and a distant (indifferent) electrode. If the potential is equal at the two points (zero potential), then no electricity flows between the two electrodes; a difference in potential between the two points is recorded as a deflection of the galvanometer. Since the potential is recorded by the galvanometer on moving paper, the electrocardiogram represents, in the language of physics, a record in which electrical

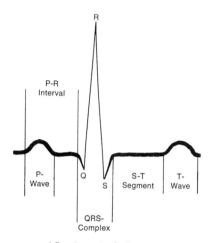

FIGURE 15. *A typical electrocardiographic lead showing the various components of the electrocardiogram.*

potential is plotted against time. In such a record zero potential is represented by a straight line, when no galvanometer deflection occurs; this is termed the *base line*. Electrical impulses traveling *toward* the exploring electrode are recorded as deflections above the base line, or positive deflections. Impulses traveling *away* from the exploring electrode are recorded below the base line as negative deflections. It is seen from figure 12 that, in the conventional electrocardiographic leads, the P-, R-, and T-waves are electropositive, and the Q- and S-waves are electronegative.

Clinical electrocardiography requires information concerning the spread of electric excitation throughout the heart, a tridimensional organ. A single electrocardiographic lead, one "viewing" electrical events from a single observation point (its exploring electrode) cannot supply more than a fraction of the needed information. Consequently it became necessary to use a series of leads which together supply the over-all picture of the electrical events in the heart. Currently used technique includes twelve electrocardiographic leads, six of which collect potential from the extremities and six from various points on the chest wall. The six

extremity leads explore the electrical activity of the heart as projected from the front surfaces of the chest; the six chest leads
explore events in the horizontal plane. Figure 16 shows diagrammatically the six extremity leads and their relationship to the heart
as the center of electrical activity. The size, duration, and direction
of the three principal deflections of the electrocardiogram in the
twelve leads provide an assessment of the mode in which electrical potential spreads throughout the heart.

The normal heart consists of two unequal ventricles: the left
ventricle has four times as much muscular tissue as the right, and
consequently generates four times as much electrical potential.
Since the left ventricle is located in the back and to the left of the
right ventricle, the over-all direction of the electrical forces generated by activation of the ventricles is *leftward* and *posteriorly*.
In diseases causing hypertrophy of the left ventricle (see chap. 6),

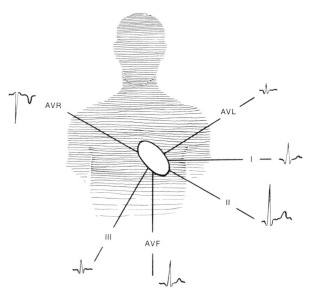

FIGURE 16. *Diagrammatic presentation of six electrocardiographic
leads, showing their shape in a normal individual and their relationship to the projection of the heart upon the front wall of the chest
(frontal plane).*

where the ratio of the two ventricles changes from 4 to 1 into 6 to 1, or 7 to 1, leftward and posterior electrical forces become even more accentuated, altering the QRS-complexes in the various leads accordingly. On the other hand, when the right ventricle hypertrophies, acquiring perhaps one-half instead of one-quarter of the musculature of the heart, the electrocardiogram shows this change by shifting the balance of forces more to the right and anteriorly.

Among other abnormalities shown by the electrocardiogram are those caused by "dead muscle." It will be shown in chapter 9 that diseases of the coronary arteries may cause damage to heart muscle by replacing living muscular tissues with softened dead tissue or with scars. This obviously affects the electrocardiogram, as the impulses have to travel around dead areas, disrupting the orderly mode of activation and introducing various irregularities into the QRS-complexes of the tracing. Furthermore, recent injury to the heart muscle produces specific changes in that the injured area acts as a "leak" in the battery whereby electric potential escapes even during the period of muscular rest. In such circumstances electrical potential is never zero, and the base line shifts away from its usual zero-point.

The most pronounced distortions of the QRS-complexes are caused by disturbances of the lower divisions of the conducting system which do not disrupt the rhythm of the heart but necessitate major "detours" and delays in the activation of the two ventricles. These disturbances are called *bundle branch blocks.*

Alterations of the P-wave of the electrocardiogram are related primarily to the size and thickness of the two atria. Such alterations permit a diagnosis of hypertrophy or enlargement of one or the other atrium. T-waves reflect the process of repolarization of the ventricles. They are influenced by a great variety of factors, and abnormal size and direction of the T-waves seldom permits a specific electrocardiographic diagnosis. Among factors altering repolarization of the ventricles are: (*a*) hypertrophy of a ventricle (in addition to the above described changes in the QRS-complexes); (*b*) areas of dead muscle; (*c*) disturbances of conduction within the ventricles; (*d*) temporary inadequacy of blood supply to the heart (ischemia); (*e*) drugs, particularly digitalis; (*f*) disturbance of salt and water metabolism in the body; and many others.

In patients with suspected disease of the coronary circulation the electrocardiogram may be normal, indicating that no major areas of dead muscle are present, and yet the physician may wish to explore the possibility that blood supply to the heart muscle is inadequate during exercise. This can often be demonstrated by recording the electrocardiogram immediately after cessation of strenuous exercise and thereby observing *temporary* alteration of the electrocardiographic complexes. This is the basis for the electrocardiographic exercise tolerance test (Master's test) consisting of walking up and down two steps at a brisk pace for one or two minutes. In normal individuals the electrocardiogram shows no change except for a faster heart rate. In those with an inadequate blood supply to the heart, specific changes may be observed.

Thus, the diagnostic uses of electrocardiography may be summarized as follows:

1) It provides an easily accessible and accurate diagnosis and analysis of all disturbances of heart rhythm.

2) It may reveal increases in the muscle mass of the left or right ventricle, providing therefore an important means of diagnosis of ventricular hypertrophy.

3) It provides important, often conclusive, evidence of major damage to the heart muscle due to coronary artery diseases.

4) It may demonstrate lesser disturbances of the circulation through the heart, including that detectable only after exercise.

5) It shows damage to the lower portions of the conducting system.

6) It may provide important information concerning the state of the atria.

7) It is an aid in the diagnosis of many other conditions in addition to those already listed: myocarditis, pericarditis, pulmonary embolism, and others. It may help in cases of gross dis-

turbances of water and electrolyte metabolism with or without involvement of the heart.

It is seen from this discussion that electrocardiography is an invaluable aid in the diagnosis of heart disease; its widespread popularity is well deserved. However, it has many important limitations which are often not appreciated, even by some physicians. The most fundamental limitation of electrocardiography is the fact that the electrical activity of the heart, which it records, is almost entirely unrelated to the function of the heart as a pump. This is best shown by observing patients change from completely normal cardiac performance into the state of severe heart failure. In many such patients, especially if no drugs have yet been administered, this transition from one to the other extreme of heart function may occur without a change in the electrocardiogram. Thus, the electrocardiogram is an essential aid in the diagnosis of some specific problems of heart disease, but is of little help in others. It should be emphasized that under certain circumstances serious heart disease may exist while the electrocardiogram is entirely normal. The reverse also occurs: heart attack may produce permanent, serious changes in the electrocardiogram which then appears grossly abnormal, and yet patients may completely recover from such attacks and lead entirely normal lives for many years thereafter.

Thus it can be concluded that the proper role of electrocardiography is to serve as a diagnostic aid to the physician, and not as a device capable in itself of making the diagnosis of heart disease.

OTHER DIAGNOSTIC EXAMINATIONS

In addition to radiographic and electrocardiographic examinations, specifically suited to the study of heart disease, there are many other tests which are readily available to the physician and are often used in individuals with heart disease or those suspected of having it. Examinations of the blood, urine, and the serological test for syphilis are usually performed on such patients as a matter of routine. In patients who have an elevated temperature, special bacteriological examinations of the blood, urine, or sputum are often made. In patients with heart failure various chemical tests of the blood are often performed to determine the level of various electrolytes, bile salts, and other body chemical substances. In recent years, measurements of some enzymes in the blood have become an important part of examination and follow-up of patients with "coronary" heart attacks, for dead muscle liberates excessive amounts of these enzymes and their level in the blood rises steeply. Various tests determining the clotting properties of the blood are frequently necessary during certain forms of treatment of heart disease (see chap. 5). Function tests of virtually every organ in the body may have to be performed in the course of a diagnostic work-up of patients who have, or are thought to have, heart disease, because major breakdown of heart function may affect many other organs of the body.

THE CARDIAC LABORATORY

The medical history, physical examination, and laboratory procedures described or enumerated in the preceding sections usually permit the expert to establish a diagnosis of heart disease with considerable accuracy. This represents the final diagnosis in many types of heart disease. There is, however, an important group of conditions involving the heart and the circulatory system in which even more detailed and specific knowledge is needed. This is particularly true in patients whose heart disease may be amenable to some type of surgical treatment. The place where highly specialized tests are performed is the "cardiac laboratory" (cardiovascular laboratory, cardiopulmonary laboratory, etc.). In such laboratories special equipment and specialized personnel are available for the performance of various tests and procedures. The expense of the equipment and the need for highly trained personnel place such procedures outside the range of the medical office, clinic, or smaller hospital. They are available in medical centers,

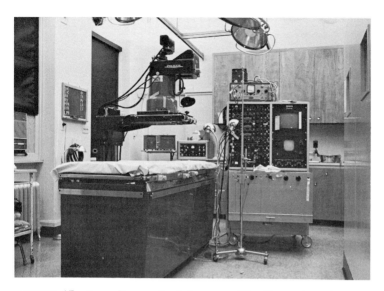

FIGURE 17. *A cardiovascular laboratory. The illustration shows as the important pieces of equipment the fluoroscopic table, to which is attached the tubular image intensifier (above the table); on top of the intensifier is the motion picture camera for cine-angiocardiography. The large console (right center) is a physiological recorder, which has two monitoring oscilloscopes and control panels to record electrocardiograms, sound records, pressure tracings, and other events occurring during the heart cycle.*

usually those associated with a cardiac-surgical program. Since technical excellence of such procedures depends upon the volume of work, most reliable work of this kind is performed in major centers, especially where it can be combined with research in heart disease. The major procedures of this category include cardiac catheterization and angiocardiography; lesser tests are vectorcardiography, phonocardiography, and others.

Cardiac catheterization was introduced in the relatively recent past; it became one of the major breakthroughs in the field of cardiology, which was duly acknowledged by awarding its originators the Nobel Prize for 1956. At first introduced as a tool for research in heart disease, cardiac catheterization soon became a method for the diagnosis of some forms of congenital heart disease. Later this technique was applied to many other forms of heart disease, and, along with angiocardiography, became the most accurate method for the study of heart diseases.

The standard cardiac catheterization consists of the introduction of a catheter (a thin tube made of a plastic material opaque to X rays) into a superficial vein in the arm or leg, and guiding it under fluoroscopic control into the right side of the heart. The most commonly used point of entry are the veins at the bend of the elbow, through which the catheter enters the venous system and floats with the stream of venous blood into the superior vena cava, the right atrium, the right ventricle, and the pulmonary artery. The catheter has holes at its tip and a connector at the other end; through it blood samples from the inside of the heart can be withdrawn for analysis; when connected with a manometric device, pressure in the heart—at the point of the opening at the tip—can be measured and recorded. Figure 18 shows a drawing of the right side of the heart superimposed on a chest X ray. The dark heavy line indicates the course of the catheter coming from the left arm into the superior vena cava, the right atrium, curving up through the tricuspid valve into the outflow tract of the right ventricle, and then through the pulmonary valve with the tip located in the pulmonary artery just above the valve. Ordinarily the catheter remains within the right side of the heart; occasionally, however, if abnormal communications exist between the two sides of the heart it may pass into its left side.

Catheterization of the right side of the heart provides certain important information which is not obtainable in any other way. It permits measurement of pressure in the right ventricle and the pulmonary artery. Abnormal elevation of pressure in them indicates pulmonary hypertension, an important condition to be discussed in chapter 15. If pressure is elevated in the right ventricle but not in the pulmonary artery, then the presence of pulmonary stenosis (obstruction at the pulmonary valve) can be deduced, for significant obstruction either raises the pressure in back of it, or lowers pressure in front of it. By taking simultaneous blood

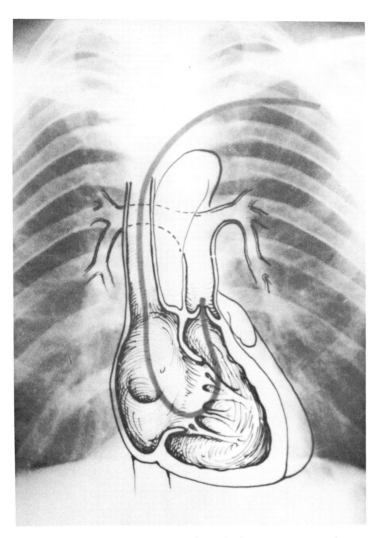

FIGURE 18. *Drawing of the right side of the heart superimposed upon a chest X ray. The black line represents the cardiac catheter with its tip located just beyond the pulmonary valve. The catheter passes through veins into the superior vena cava, the right atrium, through the tricuspid valve into the right ventricle, and then through the pulmonary valve into the pulmonary artery.*

samples from the pulmonary artery through the cardiac catheter and from a systemic artery through a needle and analyzing the oxygen content, it is possible to measure accurately the *cardiac output*. Blood samples withdrawn through the catheter from various parts of the right side of the circulation may show an unusually high content of oxygen in some samples but not in others. If this is the case then an abnormal communication within the heart can be recognized, through which highly oxygenated blood from the left side of the heart mixes with the poorly oxygenated "venous" blood; thus "shunts" can be diagnosed. In addition to the study of events in the right side of the circulation, certain limited information concerning the left side of the heart can be obtained, for by advancing the catheter into a small branch of the pulmonary artery it is possible to obtain a measurement of pressure in the left atrium.

However, advances in surgical treatment of diseases of heart valves necessitate a more detailed study of events within the left side of the heart than is possible by the standard catheterization technique. Newer approaches to cardiac catheterization now permit the entry of catheters into the left side of the heart whenever indicated. This can be done by puncturing the septum between the atria with a long needle and sliding the catheter over the needle into the left atrium, and hence into the left ventricle (*transseptal left heart catheterization*); or by directly puncturing the left lower chest wall and introducing a needle into the left ventricle; or, finally by introducing a catheter into an artery of an arm or leg and passing it against the flow of blood into the aorta, and through the aortic valve into the left ventricle (*retrograde left-sided catheterization*). The purpose of catheterization of the left side of the heart is to obtain pressure readings in the left ventricle and the left atrium which permit an evaluation of the state of the mitral and aortic valves.

Catheterization of the right side, or the left side, of the heart can be used in conjunction with many other diagnostic methods which are needed under certain special conditions. The most important procedure is the introduction through the catheter of contrast media in order to visualize its various parts in X-ray films (*angiocardiography,* to be discussed in detail). Other procedures include the introduction of harmless dyes into the right side of the heart with detector devices placed on the left side of the circulation. This procedure demonstrates shunts from the right to the left side of the circulation through abnormal communications; it may demonstrate the presence of regurgitation through one of the cardiac valves; it provides, furthermore, an alternate method for measurement of cardiac output. Special catheters can be used to detect foreign gas inhaled by the patient—this helps diagnose shunts from the left to the right side of the circulation and is more sensitive than analysis of blood samples for oxygen mentioned above. Another type of catheter has a microphone at its tip and is used to record heart sounds and heart murmurs inside the heart. Finally, in more refined evaluation of the heart function it is sometimes necessary to study responses of the circulatory system to exercise. This can be done during right-sided cardiac catheterization by performing various measurements while the patient moves stationary bicycle pedals.

Angiocardiography was originally developed as an independent test, but now is used more and more in conjunction with catheterization of the cardiovascular system. Angiocardiography, which uses X-ray equipment, consists of the introduction into the bloodstream of a liquid substance which is impenetrable to X rays and therefore appears darker on X-ray film than does any other part of the body. Modern contrast substances consist of organic compounds of iodine. As barium outlines the inside of the digestive tract while passing through its various sections, so does the contrast medium injected into the blood show the various sections of the cardiovascular system. Early angiocardiography consisted of injecting the contrast substance into the vein in the arm and taking serial X-ray films to show its passage through the heart and major vessels. Improvement in techniques brought about the rapid film changer (six films can be exposed per second) and motion picture photography of the highly intensified X-ray screen. This type of equipment and fine-grain film permit demonstration of minute details of the structure of various portions of the cardio-vascular system perfused by blood opacified with the contrast substance. However, in order to perform such studies it is not enough to inject the substance into the vein; its highest concentration is needed at the point of study. Thus the field of *selective angiocardiography* was developed, which depends on rapid injection of the opaque substance under high pressure through a cardiac catheter into the area under investigation. This method permits assessment of details inside the heart either by rapidly changing films or by cinematography. Thus one can outline each heart chamber and detect abnormal direction of blood flow, as shunts or regurgitation through incompetent valves, outline areas of obstruction, and so on. In addition to the visualization of the heart and the great arterial trunks, *selective angiography* has been applied to contrast study of specific regions of the circulation: coronary angiography provides visualization of the coronary circulation; cerebral angiography that of the circulation to the brain; renal angiography the circulation of the kidney. Virtually all arteries and veins can be visualized if the need arises to obtain such information.

Thus, angiocardiography is now usually performed in conjunction with cardiac catheterization, and many cardiac laboratories provide joint facilities for physiological measurements (cardiac catheterization) and contrast X-ray work (selective angiocardiography). However, intravenous angiocardiography still has a place in diagnosis. Its advantages are less expensive equipment and simpler technique, and thus its application is more widely available. Among simpler problems in which this method is used are: identification of unusual shadows in the chest X ray, gross identification of heart chambers, and evaluation of fluid in the pericardial sac. Certain vascular problems can also be handled with simpler equipment and the injection of a contrast medium through a needle into the area under investigation.

Cardiac catheterization and angiocardiography differ from most other diagnostic tests in that they are surgical procedures, requiring hospitalization. They carry a risk of the patient's becoming ill as a result of the procedure, and even the possibility that the patient could die from it. Such a risk, regardless of how remote, cannot be taken lightly. Therefore, it is necessary to consider carefully the benefit from the information obtained through such tests and to balance it against the risk. From the standpoint of the risk these tests can be placed on three levels: catheterization of the right side of the heart carries the lowest risk; in an experienced unit the risk is very remote indeed, especially in individuals in apparent good health. Selective angiography carries a somewhat higher risk. Catheterization of the left side of the heart carries a significantly higher risk. Thus each procedure should be performed with the full knowledge of the risk and the conviction on the part of the physician that it is justified by the benefit obtained by the patient from the more exact knowledge of his heart disease.

The complexity of the test does not automatically ensure the correctness of the information obtained. To the contrary, only a careful and critical analysis of the data can lead to acceptable diagnostic conclusions. The over-all success of these procedures is related to the careful technique, experience, and ingenuity of the members of the diagnostic team, who have to make many *ad hoc* decisions during the performance of these tests in order to select the methods most likely to produce the final answer. A high yield of correct diagnoses is likely to occur primarily in centers where a large volume of material is handled and where the team members undertake this work as their primary interest.

The following are some conditions in which cardiac catheterization and angiocardiography are often needed: (*a*) congenital heart disease, (*b*) disorders involving the pulmonary circulation, (*c*) diseases of the cardiac valves, (*d*) diseases of blood vessels suggesting localized obstruction to blood flow, (*e*) rarer and obscure forms of heart disease. In each of these groups individual cases have to be considered as to whether risks are justifiable in order to obtain important information regarding treatment and prognosis. If surgery is being considered, such tests are essential. There are, however, many situations where cardiac catheterization is indicated even if surgical treatment is not seriously considered. In younger individuals in particular there may be doubt whether cardiac disease is present or not; cardiac catheterization of the right side of the heart often provides specific answers to such questions at a negligible risk.

In addition to these major diagnostic procedures, most cardiac laboratories offer other, simpler tests which have not become part of the cardiologist's standard equipment because of their complexity on the one hand and rather limited application on the other hand. Three of these tests are discussed below.

Vectorcardiography is a variant of electrocardiography and records the same electrical events in the heart as the conventional electrocardiograph. This is a method of presenting a picture of the electrical potential of the heart in the form of loops. In physics it is customary to present various forces in the form of vectors, arrows which express the magnitude, direction, and sense of the force. The electrical potential representing the spread of activation through the heart can be shown as a series of such vectors, which together form a loop "summarizing" all forces projected in one plane. Clinical vectorcardiography deals mostly with the forces of ventricular depolarization—the QRS-loop. Loops depicting QRS-forces can be recorded automatically by a cathode-ray oscilloscope into which two electrocardiographic leads are fed simultaneously. If each lead represents one axis (head-to-foot axis, side-to-side axis, and front-to-back axis), three loops can be obtained by a combination of these axes which represent forces projected into three planes. Such vector loops are shown in figure 19.

It is clear that vectorcardiography presents the same information as electrocardiography but in a different form. There are certain theoretical advantages in vectorial presentation of electrical phenomena of the heart. The most important of these is the fact that vectorcardiography is capable of presenting these phenomena in a less distorted manner than the conventional twelve leads, for the special leads representing the three axes are arranged to be obtained from the body surface in such a manner as to make them at nearly 90 degrees to each other (orthogonal leads).

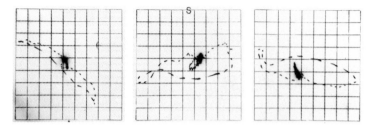

FIGURE 19. *Reproduction of a vectorcardiogram obtained by photographing the screen of an oscilloscope. Three loops are shown, each representing the QRS electrical forces in one plane. The loops are interrupted by time signals so that dot or dash represents 2/1000 second.*

Conventional electrocardiographic leads are, in contrast, subject to a great deal of distortion of electrical forces. However, from the practical standpoint, electrocardiography has the backlog of years of experience and correlation between tracings and actual findings; vectorcardiography is new and as yet limited. At this time the advantage of the more complex vectorcardiography, requiring more expensive equipment than the simpler electrocardiography, has not been established and the technique is mainly used in research and teaching.

Phonocardiography is a method of graphic registration of heart sounds and murmurs. These are recorded with acoustical filters which can selectively amplify low, medium, and high frequencies. Records are taken by placing a sensitive microphone upon the chest wall in locations where sounds and murmurs are readily heard with the stethoscope. For the purpose of timing the sound phenomena in relation to other events of the heart cycle, simultaneous recording of the electrocardiogram, pulse tracing, and, sometimes, the respiration is done on the graph.

The purpose of phonocardiography is to record the various sound phenomena originating in the heart by means of an objective method as a supplement to the description of the findings when auscultated by the human ear. Measurements of time relationship permit a much more accurate analysis of the events than is possible by auscultation alone. However, the microphone is never as sensitive as the ear; phonocardiography cannot be used in the hope of recording murmurs or sounds which are not perceived by auscultation, and the technique is no substitute for physical examination of the heart. Yet it does represent a valuable adjunct to examination and permits quantitative presentation of certain events which are an aid in diagnosis. A typical phonocardiogram is shown in figure 20.

Ballistocardiography is a method of recording motion of the body transmitted from the heart and great vessels. This method was more popular in the early 1950's than it is now, for it has since been demonstrated that the forces recorded rather crudely depict mechanical events in the circulation and can be modified by a wide variety of factors, not necessarily related to diseases of the heart. It has limited application in connection with coronary artery disease.

THE OVER-ALL APPROACH TO DIAGNOSIS

This chapter deals with the general philosophy of diagnosis of diseases of the heart and circulation. The principles and purpose of the various steps—from the patient's medical history and physical examination to the most complex procedures—have been reviewed and explained. It emphasizes the fact that diagnosis represents the thinking process of the central figure—the physician. He has to review all findings, sift the evidence, and critically evaluate the data. In the case of contradictory findings, the experienced physician will know which findings to accept and which to reject. No matter how strongly a given laboratory finding may suggest the presence of a certain disease, the diagnosis can only be made by the physician if the preponderance of other data is in accord with this. It might appear, superficially, that, with the large number of laboratory procedures now available, the diagnosis of cardiovascular diseases has been simplified. This is incorrect. Diagnostic deduction remains one of the highest endeavors in medical practice; today's more available laboratory procedures merely require broader background and better training on the part of the diagnostician.

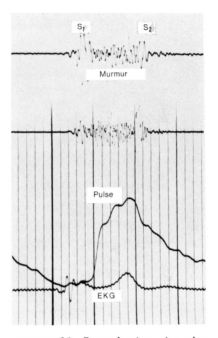

FIGURE 20. *Reproduction of a phonocardiogram. Sound tracings are shown by the two top lines. They were obtained by placing microphones on two different areas of the chest wall. The pulse curve and an electrocardiographic lead, below, are used for timing reference. The two heart sounds (S_1 and S_2) are shown by taller vibrations of the line. Between them, the space is filled with finer, irregular vibrations, representing a systolic murmur of mitral insufficiency.*

5

Treatment

Treatment of disease is often thought of in narrow terms of cure or of relief of symptoms. In diseases of the heart and circulation, treatment acquires a broader, more comprehensive meaning. To be sure, there are many instances of conventional treatment of heart diseases, for example treatment of acute diseases of the heart and acute episodes in some chronic diseases, or corrective and curative forms of cardiac surgery. However, most heart diseases constitute a chronic lifetime condition. Patients found to have heart disease look to the physician not as a dispenser of drugs, but as a personal adviser. Typical questions such as the following have to be answered: Should a child play normally with other children? Should a young man select a sedentary occupation rather than one requiring physical effort? Should an individual follow a special diet, or give up smoking? Thus, the objective of treatment is to manage day-to-day problems by means of conventional drug therapy, by diet, and by rest in bed; to consider curative procedures by medical and surgical means; to conserve the patient's reserves by regulation of his mode of living; and to anticipate and prevent problems that may arise in the future.

GENERAL PRINCIPLES

When the diagnosis of a disease of the heart is firmly established, the physician has to consider, as the next step, two further problems: the prognosis and treatment. Both prognosis and treatment acquire a much broader basis in relation to diseases of the heart than in many other fields of medicine. For example, prognosis of a given disease is often thought of in terms of the immediate outlook revolving around recovery versus death; treatment is considered a short-term action, such as drug therapy for pneumonia, or surgical treatment of appendicitis. However, the cardiologist deals mostly with problems involving long-term, life-long afflictions, rather than acute illness. Consequently, prognosis and treatment often become part of the same mental process, concerned with the question: Can the outlook for the future be modified by treatment? Thus the physician treating heart disease often has to undertake the role of a consultant who advises his patient in many aspects other than the heart and helps him plan his life.

In order to exemplify this, let us suppose that a cardiologist has completed his diagnostic evaluation of a patient and has established the presence of a disease of the heart. His choice of courses of action include the following:

1) He may permit the patient to live a normal and totally unrestricted life without any treatment.

2) He may regulate the patient's mode of living as to activities, diet, and habits, but still elect not to recommend any active long-term treatment.

3) He may treat the patient by drugs and by regulation of his mode of living, but let him engage in his customary occupation.

4) He may find it necessary, in spite of active treatment, to recommend retraining of the patient to a more suitable, less strenuous, or even sedentary, occupation, or may advise retirement.

5) He may instigate short-term medical or surgical treatment in the hospital.

There are, of course, many other possibilities, but it is well to appreciate that broad considerations affecting the entire life of a patient may have to be undertaken in dealing with heart disease. In the discussion that follows some of the general principles involved in cardiac therapy will be briefly presented.

DRUG THERAPY

A great many drugs affect the heart and circulation directly or indirectly, but there are a few key "cardiac drugs" which play the major part in treatment of heart disease.

Digitalis, the oldest drug in continuous usage, is an active extract from the leaves of foxglove. Used originally as a brew, it was then used as a powder derived from dried foxglove leaves. Such powder is now carefully standardized by testing its action on animals; however, several forms of purified active ingredients derived from this plant are now available and have to some extent replaced the powdered leaf. The purified compounds, digitalis "glycosides," are more stable, and, like other currently used drugs, have their dosages expressed in terms of weight rather than animal action. Digitalis has many actions on the various functions of the heart and circulation and is one of the most powerful drugs (and poisons) available. Two principal properties of this drug constitute the basis of its use in patients with heart disease:

1) Digitalis and its derivatives act by delaying and partially blocking the conduction of impulses from the atria to the ventricles through the conducting system. This property of the drug is especially useful in atrial fibrillation (see chap. 7), where too many impulses are sent from the atria to the ventricles, leading to excessive ventricular rates. Digitalis is capable, by its blocking action, of slowing down the ventricular rate to a desired level, which usually results in dramatic improvement of the patient's condition.

2) Digitalis increases the strength of ventricular contraction, thereby being a basic drug for treatment of heart failure.

Both actions of digitalis are related to the metabolism of the heart muscle cells, particularly the transfer of ions through the cell membrane. In order to obtain the desired effect it is necessary to "saturate" the body with digitalis, giving large amounts of it until the desired effect is obtained; afterwards small doses are regularly administered in order to replace the quantity of digitalis excreted or destroyed by the body. Too large doses of digitalis may cause many undesirable symptoms, such as loss of appetite, nausea, vomiting, and irregularities of heart action. Overdoses of digitalis may endanger the patient's life.

Quinidine is derived from the bark of the tropical cinchona tree and is related to quinine. Its principal action is to reduce or eliminate overactive impulses within the heart which can be responsible for the premature beats and paroxysms of rapid heart action. Quinidine is hence used primarily in the treatment of arrhythmias (chap. 7). Unlike the long and sustained action of digitalis, quinidine acts quickly and for short periods of time; consequently, it has to be administered several times a day. It is used to terminate such arrhythmias as atrial fibrillation, flutter, and atrial and ventricular tachycardias (see chap. 7); in smaller doses it can be used to prevent recurrence of these arrhythmias and to treat recurrent minor irregularities, such as premature beats.

Procaine amide (known also under its trade name of Pronestyl) is a drug originally used as a local anesthetic (a derivative of the popular Novocain), which has also been found to have important properties of eliminating some irregular and abnormal heart actions. Its action resembles somewhat that of quinidine: both affect the metabolism of heart muscle cells by reducing their responsiveness to stimuli. Procaine amide, however, differs from quinidine in that it has a more powerful action in the treatment and prevention of arrhythmias originating in the ventricles, but a weaker action in atrial arrhythmias. This drug, like quinidine, is administered in divided doses throughout the day, or, in urgent situations, can be given intravenously with caution.

Diuretic drugs have the property of eliminating excess fluid, with particular effectiveness against fluid accumulated in the organism as a result of heart failure. They include a large number of agents; the older diuretics have more historical than practical importance; among those are derivatives of caffeine (hence coffee and tea are weak diuretics). The introduction of modern diuretics revolutionized the treatment of heart failure by virtually eliminating the much dreaded "dropsy." The most important currently used diuretics include the following: (*a*) organic compounds of mercury (meralluride—Mercuhydrin, mercaptomerin—Thiomerin), which are most effectively given by injection; (*b*) derivatives of the chemical compound thiazide, including chlorthiazide (Diuril) and a great variety of related compounds; and (*c*) drugs inhibiting enzymes and hormones related to the process of water elimination (diamox, lactospirone —Aldactone).

These drugs affect the excretory function of the kidneys in various ways, increasing the elimination of sodium and water from the blood, which in turn is replaced from the waterlogged tissues of the patient with edema. Mercurial compounds, administered by injection, are given at intervals of days or weeks, often only when needed. The other two types of diuretics are given in tablet form either daily and continuously, or several times a week according to specific schedules. The most effective index of action of diuretics on the one hand, or need for the diuretic on the other hand, is rapid change in body weight: loss of five to ten pounds often follows a single injection of a diuretic; sudden weight gain usually indicates that such treatment is needed.

Nitroglycerin is a drug with the property of relieving chest pain due to inadequate blood supply to the heart (angina pectoris, coronary insufficiency). Its action is not entirely understood; according to some it dilates coronary arteries, improving blood supply to the heart; others believe that nitroglycerin reduces the work of the heart, thereby decreasing the demands for augmented coronary blood flow. It is most effective when administered under the tongue; tablets of nitroglycerin dissolve promptly in the saliva and are rapidly absorbed; relief is instantaneous. Its duration, however, is very short and the drug is useless when given at regular intervals; its prime purpose is to terminate an attack of pain when it occurs, or to prevent an anticipated attack under circumstances when such an attack usually takes place. Once the action of the drug is over, often in a matter of minutes, it has no further effect whatsoever. When it is needed therefore nitroglycerin may be taken many times a day. Another agent with an identical action is amyl nitrite, a liquid with a sharp and penetrating smell which is ordinarily inhaled; it is seldom used nowadays, for nitroglycerin is much easier to administer. There are a large number of drugs related to nitroglycerin (nitrites) which theoretically act similarly and, because of long-lasting effects in tablet form, can be used at regular intervals rather than during attacks. Such drugs are widely used, and yet their effectiveness is still a matter of controversy among investigators: some more critical work indicates that the action of these drugs in preventing attacks of chest pain is entirely unproved.

Anticoagulant agents are among widely used drugs in heart diseases, but are totally unrelated to heart action. These drugs interfere with the normal mechanism of blood clotting; their objective is to prevent blood clotting within the heart and blood vessels—a common complication of some forms of heart disease.

There are two types of anticoagulant agents: those acting directly on the clotting mechanism by interrupting the chain of chemical events leading to the clotting of blood, both inside the body and in the test tube; the other group acts primarily upon the liver and prevents the formation of one of the essential substances in the process of clotting, but has no direct effect upon blood clotting in the test tube.

The first category of drugs is represented by *heparin,* a powerful substance normally present in the body. Heparin has to be given by injection and has the disadvantage of having a short-lived effect so that it has to be administered more than once a day. This agent is therefore most suitable for short-term treatment. The second category of anticoagulant drugs includes a variety of chemical agents related to the compound coumarin— a substance contained in clover leaves—and other, similarly acting synthetic drugs. These agents act more slowly and are effective in tablet form, and are therefore the first choice in long-term therapy.

Since anticoagulants tamper with an important defense mechanism of the body, treatment has to be carefully assessed so that clotting within vessel walls is prevented and yet no danger of internal hemorrhage or excessive bleeding from minor cuts is introduced. This can be done by periodic tests of the effectiveness of treatment. When heparin is used, direct measurement of clotting time of the blood outside the body is the index of its efficacy. With coumarin derivatives and related drugs, the *prothrombin time test* provides such an index.

The use of anticoagulant drugs is rather tricky and carries a definite risk of hemorrhage because blood tests are imperfect in revealing the exact effect of the drugs, and because they cannot be performed daily over a long period of time, but rather weekly or monthly. The most widely accepted use of these drugs is in the prevention of clot formation and extension of existing clots in the venous system. These drugs have also received wide application in diseases of the coronary arteries both in the acute stage of myocardial infarction and in its chronic form. Here, however, anticoagulant therapy is the subject of considerable controversy, since some authorities believe that the effectiveness of these drugs in the prevention of clot formation within the heart and the coronary arteries is neither dependable nor consistent enough to justify the risk of their administration. These drugs are now used according to the individual preferences of physicians.

In addition to the drugs discussed in the preceding sections, the physician uses a great many other drugs in the treatment of diseases of the heart and circulation. Sedatives and tranquilizers are important in controlling some symptoms and anxiety of the patient; pain-killers and sleeping tablets are frequently needed. Antibiotics play an important part in the treatment of infections of the heart itself or of other organs. Drugs affecting the autonomic nervous system have a wide application in some disorders of the heart and blood vessels. Hypotensive drugs are capable of controlling high blood pressure; they will be discussed later (chap. 11).

DIETARY THERAPY

Treatment of heart disease by special diets has been used widely for many years; however, most of such treatment was based on nonscientific, fad-like approaches. It is now generally believed that there is no scientific evidence to suggest that diet can, under ordinary circumstances, alter the course of heart disease. Yet there are three areas in which dietary treatment supplements other forms of therapy:

1) A general low calorie diet is very important for those patients in whom overweight is a problem. Excess body weight imposes an additional work load upon the circulation. In patients with reduced cardiac reserve this added work load may be a factor in bringing about or perpetuating heart failure. As a general rule, a chronic cardiac patient should aim at being below figures obtained from the average weight tables rather than at, or above, them.

2) Low salt diet is an important part of management of patients who have tendencies to fluid retention. Salt, or rather its component the kation sodium, facilitates accumulation of fluid in the tissues. In patients with moderate tendencies for water retention strict observance of low sodium diet will reduce, or even eliminate, the need for the administration of diuretic drugs. In more advanced cases, both diuretic therapy and salt restriction are needed to control fluid retention. The degree of salt restriction in the diet varies considerably. The average normal diet contains between 10 and 20 grams of salt per day; mild restriction of salt in the diet would reduce this figure to 3 to 5 grams of salt per 24 hours; moderate restriction cuts the salt to 1 to 3 grams; and severe restriction to below 1 gram. In rare cases it may be necessary to restrict the salt to less than 0.2 grams per day. Low salt diet is an important adjunct in the treatment of heart failure. Since more strict diet reduces the need

for diuretic drugs, and vice-versa, plans may be designed to suit the individual patient's preferences in those cases where it is not necessary to use the full extent of both measures. In addition to treatment of heart failure, low salt diet is sometimes used also as an adjunct to treatment of hypertension.

3) Low fat diet has been in the limelight of medical and lay press alike. Its use is based on some epidemiological observations concerning the low incidence of atherosclerosis and the resulting heart attacks in populations fed on a low fat or low animal fat diet. The role of the dietary factor in the prevention of atherosclerotic complications will be discussed in chapter 10. It may be stated here that many authorities believe that it has not been demonstrated beyond reasonable doubt that such dietary restriction lessens the probability of the progression of atherosclerosis, and feel that a rigid adherence to such diets may not now be justifiable. On the other hand, however, some authorities recommend such diets for those who have had "heart attacks" and even feel that a general revision of the standard American diet, rich in animal fat, may be justifiable for the entire population. This controversy will have to be resolved by further research; many centers in the country are now conducting long-term observations concerning this relationship.

REGULATION OF ACTIVITIES

The question as to how active a patient with heart disease should be imposes many problems. On the one hand, it is obvious that a poorly performing heart can benefit from rest; on the other hand, exercise enhances the over-all fitness of the individual. The physician caught on the horns of this dilemma has to decide and judge the merits in each individual case. The range of restriction of the patient's activities varies greatly, as has already been mentioned.

The most rigid restriction imposed on patients is *complete bed rest*. This is used ordinarily only for limited periods of time and has specific application in the acute afflictions of the heart.

In such cases it can be assumed that even the slightest activity could either interfere with the healing of an acute damage to the heart, or enhance an undesirable and avoidable complication. In a sense, complete bed rest is analogous to placing a fractured extremity in a plaster cast. Among the conditions requiring complete rest are: acute myocardial infarction, acute myocarditis, and acute rheumatic carditis. In many other situations rest is desirable, but less rigid enforcement is acceptable. Modified rest takes the form of the patient's dividing his time between lying in bed and sitting in a bedside chair, with privileges of using the bathroom. Complete bed rest has specific disadvantages:

1) Complete rest lasting more than two weeks may produce some undesirable metabolic changes in cells and organs.

2) Lack of exercise may interfere with some vital action of organs other than the heart.

3) Rest enhances the formation of clots in the veins and may therefore facilitate the production of dangerous emboli.

4) Rest may produce anxiety and emotional stress in the patient.

These disadvantages compel the thoughtful physician to consider the pro's and con's in each patient before enforcing such treatment. Furthermore, it should be appreciated that in the strict physiological sense complete rest is unattainable: while resting, the individual cannot remain in the "basal" state; food consumption increases demands upon the circulation; furthermore, the very restrictions imposed on the patient often cause emotional unrest which may tax heavily the circulation. For these and some other reasons, many acute manifestations of chronic heart disease, such as the onset of heart failure, are treated with a minimum period of rest necessitated by symptoms.

In the presence of chronic heart disease physicians are often guided by symptoms in recommending restriction of activities. Thus, if shortness of breath or chest pain is repeatedly brought on by a certain activity, the patient may be advised to limit himself to activities less than those producing these symptoms.

Since the tolerance of effort varies widely in cardiac patients, some may be compelled to limit themselves to slow walks, while others merely give up such luxuries as sports and strenuous recreational activities. There are, of course, situations where the rules of self-regulation by symptoms may be ill advised, and the physician has to restrict patients more than the activities easily tolerated by them.

While restriction of activities may play a part in proper management of heart disease, reasonable exercise may also be important for the patient. In those patients who have no acute cardiac problems and whose tolerance for exercise is good, some forms of exercise may be of benefit to them, for there is reasonable scientific evidence that general physical fitness enhances well-being in general and may benefit the circulation in particular.

PREVENTIVE MEASURES
AND REHABILITATION

Preventive measures and rehabilitation, particularly directed at younger individuals with heart disease, are an important part of the management of heart disease. The objective of such measures is to protect individuals from the various external influences which could cause progression of the disease, to try to preserve proper function of the heart as long as possible, and to prevent complications. Among such preventive measures are the regulation of such habits as the use of tobacco and alcohol; the encouragement of weight reduction; moderate exercise, when permissible (see above); the prevention of infection (particularly rheumatic fever and endocarditis) by antibiotics.

Rehabilitation includes retraining individuals for less strenuous occupations. In dealing with school-age individuals it is important to advise them in the selection of vocations less likely to affect their heart condition adversely in the future. Other rehabilitative measures may consist of various forms of physical and occupational therapy in patients laid up with serious forms of heart disease, both during the illness and after recovery;

treatment of strokes; and other common complications of heart disease.

SURGICAL TREATMENT
OF CARDIOVASCULAR DISEASE

Cardiac surgery represents one of the most dramatic developments in the recent history of medical science. It has captured the imagination of the medical profession and the lay public alike, and has acquired an aura of sensationalism, which, on occasion, has colored the approach to it. It should be obvious, however, that only a sober "second look" can bring this field into the proper perspective.

Surgical treatment of diseases of the heart and vessels falls into three general categories:

CURATIVE SURGERY

This is a form of surgical treatment in which a status comparable with that of a normal individual can be brought about; in other words, a complete cure is accomplished by the operation. Two operations on the vascular system have withstood the test of time and fall firmly into this category: closure of patent ductus arteriosus and repair of coarctation of the aorta. These operations successfully cure two serious congenital defects. Among operations within the heart, two procedures aided by use of open-heart techniques can be placed tentatively in this category: the repair of simple atrial septal defects and of smaller ventricular septal defects associated with normal pressure in the pulmonary artery. These operations are relatively new; thus far they appear to be curative; however, long-term follow-up is not yet available.

CORRECTIVE SURGERY

This category includes most currently successful operations upon the cardiovascular system: surgical treatment here improves an existing abnormality, but normal conditions cannot be entirely reestablished. Such treatment in many cases approximates the first group. *Almost* normal relationships may be established and for practical purposes the patient is close to being cured; in other cases a greater or lesser degree of improvement may be noted. There are, of course, cases where the operation produces little or no improvement. "Corrective" surgery includes all types of operations on heart valves (including their replacement), and on congenital malformations other than those listed in the first category.

PALLIATIVE SURGERY

In this group of procedures the original defect or abnormality of the heart or blood vessels is left unchanged, but the operation is aimed at removal of some of the undesirable consequences of it. This includes conditions for which no operation is available, or those where an operation may be performed with more safety at a later time. In this category one can name the various shunting operations (such as the famous Blalock–Taussig "blue-baby" operation) and procedures designed at restriction of excessive blood flow to the lungs.

The major breakthrough in the field of cardiac surgery came with the development of satisfactory and safe artificial heart–lung machines. Surgery of the heart was the "last frontier" of operative treatment because of the difficult problem of how to operate upon the pump without disrupting the circulation to vital organs. The introduction of the finger and instruments into chambers of the heart permitted some limited relief of obstruction of heart valves. Only when it became possible to operate under open vision with sufficient time available to repair defects and deformities could cardiac surgery attempt more complex problems. The heart–lung machine, developed as a temporary substitute for the pumping action of the heart, can now maintain the circulation through the brain, the heart, and other vital organs for several hours, if necessary. The mechanics of such artificial perfusion of the body with blood consists of draining venous blood into a series of tubes outside the body, of oxygenating it and eliminating carbon dioxide ("artificial lung"), and of pumping the blood back into the arterial system in such a way as to deliver a normal, or almost normal, amount of blood under customary pressure. This is usually done by inserting cannulae into the two venae cavae to drain the venous blood, by exposing the blood to oxygen or air in large flat surfaces (disks), by bubbling oxygen through the blood, or by interposing a membrane between the blood and oxygen, and then by passing it through a motor-driven pump into a large artery in the leg. Such a circuit is represented in diagrammatic form in figure 21. The blood from the artificial pump then flows in the aorta opposite to the usual direction (upward) and perfuses the coronary circulation and brain along with other areas. The heart can then be opened, stopped if necessary, and subjected to surgical repairs. Early problems with the artificial heart–lung machine revolved mostly around the handling of blood outside the body without damaging the cells or making it clot. Furthermore, the additional circuit required large amounts of "priming" blood, as many as 15 pints of it at times, whereby patients were subjected to massive blood transfusions. These and other problems concerning the mechanics of maintaining proper pressure and flow during the perfusion and of not interfering with various biochemical adjustments in the body caused years of work and delays until satisfactory pumps were perfected.

Today, open-heart surgery aided by near-perfect pump-oxygenators can be performed in many institutions with great safety, approaching the ideal point where operations with the use of the pump-oxygenator carry no greater risk than any type of surgical operation. However, the great complexity of the process of artificial perfusion and the many problems of caring for the patient before and after the perfusion impose great demands upon the medical personnel over and above the surgical skill of operating on the heart itself, so that specially trained teams are necessary to undertake this type of procedure.

The complexity and expense of open-heart surgery make it

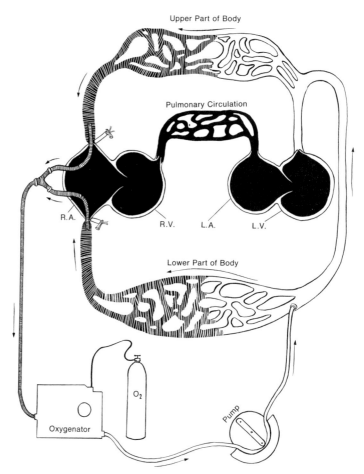

FIGURE 21. *Diagrammatic presentation of the artificial circulation used during open-heart surgery. Venous (deoxygenated) blood is shown by shaded areas, oxygenated blood by white areas. Sections of the circulation shown in black represent the areas bypassed by this artificial circuit, which can be open for repairs. All the blood returning from the superior vena cava and inferior vena cava is withdrawn and channeled through an oxygenator and a pump, then delivered into the arterial system. The blood is prevented from returning into the heart by the aortic valve. (Abbreviations: R.A., right atrium; R.V., right ventricle; L.A., left atrium; L.V., left ventricle.)*

mandatory that cases be selected with great care. The exact diagnosis is usually established by cardiac catheterization, sometimes with angiocardiography. In each case it is then necessary to weigh the risks of operating against the risks of not operating. This process of balancing pro's and con's of the operation is often expressed in the following terms: (*a*) risk of not surviving the operation; (*b*) risk of obtaining either no improvement at all, or an insignificant degree of improvement; (*c*) the cost of the operation and the loss of time and income (if the patient is the breadwinner of a family). On the other side, the physician has to estimate the projected course of the disease if not operated upon, in terms of life expectancy, disability in the future, and the development of preventable complications which may render the case inoperable in the future. Many other factors come into consideration in the decision-making. For example, a curative operation which can be performed at a very low risk is justifiable in an individual who has no symptoms and appears to be in perfect health. On the other hand, operations with higher risks and uncertain results should be contemplated only in patients with considerable disability and definite danger signs.

It should be pointed out that the process of balancing respective risks can only be considered a rough approximation. Surgical mortality should be related to a specific institution, for there are wide ranges of skills and experience in various units, with great differences in risks and results from hospital to hospital. The life expectancy and projected future disability of the un-operated patient is also only a matter of crude conjecture because of the many factors that come into play, and because of the inadequate mortality statistics concerning congenital heart disease. However, regardless of how imperfect this process of balancing risks may be, it provides the only reasonable approach to the selection of patients for cardiac surgery. It represents also a way to avoid the temptation, present in the physician and patient alike, to undertake surgical treatment of a given defect for the sole reason that such an operation has been developed!

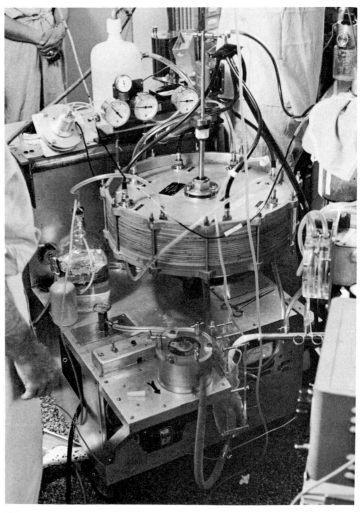

FIGURE 22. *The artificial heart-lung machine: the illustration shows the Bramson–Osborn–Gerbode membrane pump oxygenator. The large drum is the oxygenator, in which layers of blood come into contact with layers of oxygen, the two being separated by a thin permeable membrane. This oxygenator uses the same principle of oxygenation as the human lung. The small cylinder attached to the base of the machine is the pump.*

6

Performance of the Heart and Its Failure

Like most engines, the heart ordinarily uses only a fraction of its power. The heart and circulation are taxed most heavily during strenuous exercise, when the reserve power of the heart is called upon. Individuals whose physical performance is unusually heavy, such as athletes, need a stronger heart than persons with more sedentary habits. The heart of an athlete responds to this need by growth of the heart muscle, similar to the powerful weightlifter's biceps. However, in certain forms of heart disease the energy of the heart is wasted because its work is increased, not by larger body demands, but by pumping blood at higher pressure or by ejecting excessive amounts of blood. In response to this increased work load the heart muscle grows excessively, beyond the limits of the athlete's heart growth. With such overgrowth the efficiency of the engine begins to suffer, the reserve power of the heart is encroached upon, and the heart performs under adverse conditions. When the point is reached that the human body has to adapt itself to a reduced "circulatory budget," then the term "heart failure" is applied to the resulting symptoms.

In spite of its ominous connotations, the term "heart failure" does not represent the fatal, terminal stage of heart disease, but is used merely to indicate a state in which there is a significant impairment of the performance of the heart as a pump. Another

97

term used synonymously with heart failure is "cardiac insufficiency." A third one, "decompensation," is used in certain forms of chronic diseases of the heart and will be referred to later in the chapter. Heart failure signifies to the physician a set of symptoms and signs appearing in patients whose hearts are incapable of maintaining adequate circulatory functions in relation to the body demands. Such conditions may exist temporarily or permanently. As a general rule, heart failure represents a stage in the process of the deterioration of cardiac performance resulting most commonly from long-standing overwork ("overload" of the heart) in the course of certain forms of heart disease.

CARDIAC PERFORMANCE AND CARDIAC WORK LOAD

In order to better understand the relationship between cardiac performance in health and in disease it is necessary to turn back to normal responses to exercise, discussed in chapter 3. It has been indicated that during the most strenuous possible exercise by an average individual the demands of oxygen (its fuel) increase to a level *sixteen times* the minimal, basal requirements. In order to support these high demands the heart has to increase its work load about *four times*. It is obvious that at rest the average heart uses one-quarter of its maximum capacity; the remaining three-quarters represents its *reserve*. Under normal living conditions many demands are made upon this cardiac reserve. The work load of the heart has to be considered in terms of its activities within the 24-hour period. The lowest level of work load occurs in an individual placed on bed rest, but even such individuals call upon their cardiac reserve, as explained in chapter 5, so that the net work load over the 24-hour period should be somewhere between 110 and 120 percent of basal value. An individual leading a mostly sedentary life may not tax his heart more than to a level of 200 percent of basal work at any given time; his 24-hour average may be between 120 and 150 percent. Physical laborers may use up their reserves at a rate averaging 150 to 200 percent of basal work load. Trained athletes have still higher averages, although they make very strenuous efforts for only brief periods during a 24-hour day. The heart muscle adapts itself to the work load of each individual; the athlete and the laborer have heavier hearts than the sedentary worker. Increase in thickness and weight of the heart is due to the large size of each muscle fiber, a process called *hypertrophy* of the heart. Thus, slight degrees of hypertrophy occur under normal conditions in response to work habits of some individuals.

In contrast to the hypertrophy due to higher demands and utilization of cardiac reserve, there are abnormal conditions caused by heart disease in which cardiac work load is increased *without* higher demands imposed by increases of body activity. This represents the pathological (abnormal) overload of the heart, one of the most important processes operating in cardiac disease, which may lead to pathological hypertrophy of the heart, much more severe than the physiological hypertrophy of the athlete. To exemplify this mechanism one can consider a simple type of cardiac overload: hypertension. Suppose an individual has an arterial blood pressure of 240 mm. Hg, twice the normal average level, and maintains this pressure throughout 24 hours. Inasmuch as cardiac work consists of pressure times output (see chap. 3), the basal cardiac work of this patient is twice that of a normal individual. However, this patient still calls upon his cardiac reserve to perform various activities: thus, a sedentary hypertensive patient with a basal work load of 200 percent of a normal individual would have a 24-hour average of 240 percent instead of 120 percent, and a hypertensive laborer would have an average of 340 percent of the normal basal work load instead of 170 percent. These figures show the severe increase in cardiac work load in some forms of heart disease— an increase most significant because it works continuously, and therefore has to be added to the usual temporary work increments.

Hypertrophy produced by this type of cardiac overload is, as mentioned, much more pronounced than the physiologic slight hypertrophy of heavy workers. It does help the heart to carry the larger work load; it *compensates* for the excessive work. Such patients, when otherwise in good health, may actually show a normal response to exercise; they are still capable of increasing the cardiac output to four times the basal level. Thus, if the normal basal work load is taken as 100 percent and the normal individual is capable of increasing cardiac work load up to 400 percent, a fully compensated hypertensive patient has a range from 200 percent (his basal level) to 800 percent. This upper level, however, is an exception; more often than not hypertrophy compensates only partly for the increased basal work load, and patients begin to lose their reserve. Top cardiac performance may become limited to 200 or 300 percent of their basal work levels. Capacity for the performance of work becomes limited as the reserve decreases. This is a state of partial compensation. As the process advances, the point is reached where cardiac reserve is incapable of carrying out an adequate function with minor activities or even at rest without rearranging its mode of operation. This is the stage of *decompensation,* or heart failure.

The process of increased work load, just described, is an important, though not the only, mechanism producing heart failure. Increased work load involves each cardiac ventricle separately, but it may involve both together. Consequently, hypertrophy, partial compensation, and failure may affect the left ventricle, the right ventricle, or both ventricles. There are two principal types of ventricular overloads, in line with the formula for cardiac work: either the pressure is increased or the output is increased. It is customary to refer to the types of overload as *pressure overload* and *volume overload,* respectively.

Pressure overload occurs when the systolic pressure in the cardiac ventricle becomes significantly elevated. This is the result of an increased resistance to flow (see chap. 3). The two possible points of increased resistance are:

1) Resistance may occur at the outflow from the ventricle in the form of *stenosis* (narrowing) of a semilunar valve, or the areas below or above the valves.

2) Excessive resistance may occur at the terminal point of the arterial reservoir—the arterioles (the stopcock; see fig. 13); this occurs in hypertension of the systemic or the pulmonary circulation.

Pressure overload is usually considered significant and likely to cause the chain of events described above, starting with compensatory hypertrophy, if the systolic pressure in the left ventricle increases by more than 50 percent (from 120 to 180 mm. Hg), or if it at least doubles in the right ventricle (from 25 to 50 mm. Hg). Usually pressures much higher than those are the cause of chronic heart disease.

Volume overload occurs when an excessive amount of blood is ejected from a cardiac ventricle. This, of course, has to occur continuously, for temporary increases of cardiac output with exercise represent normal responses. Upon rare circumstances such conditions exist in relation to the entire heart, when increased demands cause an abnormally high output of the entire heart (high output states). However, the commonest forms of volume overload occur when the increased ejection is due to a disease process which wastefully deflects the blood from the normal circulatory pathways. This occurs in two conditions:

1) Cardiac shunts, communications between two sides of the heart, usually due to congenital defects in which blood may needlessly recirculate through the lungs.

2) Regurgitation through incompetent valves when the ventricle has to eject much more blood than is needed for body demands because of its loss due to backflow through "leaky" valves.

As in pressure overload, the amount of increased work load from volume overload has to be rather large: an ejection of blood of twice the normal amount is likely to produce hypertrophy; an overload may be considerably higher than this, for large congenital shunts often increase blood flow to the lungs four times; similarly, severe valve insufficiency may lead to such a degree of regurgitation that only 25 percent of the ejected blood is utilized, while 75 percent is regurgitated, which also increases work load four times.

Thus, cardiac hypertrophy can be defined as a compensatory growth of the heart muscle which occurs in response to increased work load of the heart independent of the demands of the body. Such hypertrophy occurs in two forms:

1) Hypertrophy associated with a normal size of the cavity of the overloaded ventricle—*concentric hypertrophy.* This type of hypertrophy occurs usually in the presence of pressure overload.

2) Hypertrophy connected with enlargement of the cavity of the affected ventricle—*excentric hypertrophy,* or hypertrophy with dilatation of the heart. Excentric hypertrophy occurs more often in the presence of volume overload, but enlargement of cavity may also occur in the late stages of pressure overload.

In general, dilatation of the ventricle or of any chamber of the heart represents an undesirable event in the course of heart disease. The clinician recognizes dilatation as *cardiac enlargement,* detectable by X rays or other methods of examination; it is considered as evidence of "strain" of the heart. In heart failure dilatation of the heart is usually present and may be severe.

CARDIAC FAILURE

Thus cardiac failure can be considered an end segment of a continuous process that develops in response to overloading of the heart. Hypertrophy and, in part, dilatation help carry this load at first without major loss of cardiac performance, utilizing cardiac reserve. Such processes of compensation may last months or years; in fact, sometimes compensation of an overloading lesion may last a lifetime, so that the patient never enters the stage of failure. However, in most cases, sooner or later the process of compensation becomes inadequate and the stage of heart failure develops. As stated, failure may affect each ventricle separately or may involve both ventricles. The failing ventricles are dilated, filled with excess blood, because the heart cannot empty itself normally. Furthermore, the ejection of blood in the failing heart requires higher than normal filling pressure: the diastolic pressure of the failing heart and the corresponding atrial pressure behind it rise to abnormal levels; instead of the normal level of 2 to 8 mm. Hg, one can find pressures of 25 or 30 mm. Hg. In spite of the higher filling pressure, the failing ventricle finds it harder to eject blood and the cardiac output falls below the normal level. As a consequence, basal tissue requirements have to be met from reserve stores of oxygen in the blood; thus venous blood returning from the tissue is no longer 75 percent saturated with oxygen but only 50 or 60 percent. When an individual in heart failure exercises, cardiac output rises less than normal, if at all. Further reserves have to be tapped by extracting a still higher fraction of oxygen from the blood. In some such individuals even minor activities cause the oxygen content of venous blood to drop close to zero. As explained in chapter 4, the individual who performs close to the maximum capabilities of his circulatory system is aware of respiratory effort by experiencing shortness of breath. Circulatory inefficiency also manifests itself by a feeling of complete exhaustion associated with slight effort.

Changes in the body associated with heart failure are very profound indeed. Failure of the left ventricle increases pressure in the left atrium. The blood is "dammed" behind the failing ventricle, which is incapable of emptying itself properly. High left atrial pressure causes increased pressure in the pulmonary circulation and right side of the heart. As a consequence of increased quantities of the dammed, stagnant blood in the lungs and the higher pressure in the pulmonary circulation, the lungs become heavier and stiffer—a phenomenon called *congestion of the lungs* (pulmonary congestion), which is primarily responsible for the various forms of shortness of breath described in chapter 4. Such congestion of the lungs can also be recognized by the physician on physical examination of the lungs and in the chest X ray.

In addition to the consequences of left ventricular failure upon the lungs and respiration, the low cardiac output, which occurs in left ventricular as well as in right ventricular failure, produces another chain of events. The body tissues compelled to subsist on a "low-oxygen budget" try to help their economy by reducing blood flow to less essential areas in order to conserve blood supply for the more vital organs. Among organs suffering from this economy drive are the kidneys, which ordinarily have a very abundant blood supply. The reduction of blood flow through the kidneys is, however, a mixed blessing because it causes an undesirable interference with the process of salt and water excretion in the kidneys. In addition, the adrenal glands and the pituitary gland, which produce hormones regulating salt and water content in the body, receive distress signals from the failing circulatory system, which leads to an increase in their production of these hormones. A combination of the two factors, reduction of blood flow through the kidneys and increased production of salt-and-water hormones, cause the well-known tendency for water retention in the tissues that develops in heart failure. This is aided by still another factor: increased pressure in the right atrium due to *right* ventricular failure, which, in turn, raises the pressure in the systemic veins and the capillary system, thereby driving more water into the tissues. As tissues become waterlogged by deposition of fluid in spaces between cells (*extracellular space*), there is a rise in the total amount of blood circulating in the body (*increased blood volume*). Gradually all tissues become waterlogged, and, when the quantity of excess fluid reaches sizeable proportions, usually in excess of 10 pounds, then fluid accumulation becomes visible in the form of swollen feet, ankles, legs, and the lower part of the back. This is called *edema* (puffy swelling of subcutaneous tissues). Excess fluid may also be deposited in many other loose tissues of the body, particularly the serous membranes (membranes lining the cavities of the chest and abdomen). Accumulation of edema fluid in the chest (*pleural effusion*) may further aggravate breathing difficulties by compressing the already congested lungs. The abdominal cavity can accommodate large quantities of fluid (*ascites*), producing discomfort by pressure on various structures. Furthermore, fluid may also accumulate between the two layers of the pericardium (*pericardial effusion*), compounding cardiac difficulties. Finally, excess fluid may accumulate *within* important organs, producing undesirable and even dangerous interference with their function. The most dreaded complication of heart failure is the accumulation of fluid in the lungs—pulmonary edema—which produces a serious, often fatal, form of dyspnea (see chap. 4).

It is seen from the above discussion that the development of heart failure activates a vicious cycle: cardiac performance is impaired, whereby fluid accumulation develops; excess fluid in various tissues and organs further increases cardiac difficulties; failure is aggravated; and so on. It is now clear why the introduction of powerful diuretics for the control of fluid accumulation (dropsy) has revolutionized treatment of cardiac failure (see chap. 5).

What are the causes of heart failure? One of the common causes—the end process of chronic overloading of the heart—has been discussed in detail. If the cause of the overloading is progressive, such as increasing elevation of blood pressure or progressive narrowing of a valve orifice, then sooner or later the compensatory hypertrophy of the heart muscle will reach the point of diminishing efficiency, reduction of performance, and failure. This is caused by the fact that oxygen supply to the heart muscle becomes more difficult as the muscle becomes thicker. However, in most cases such a progression of the increased work load does not take place: the cardiac overload on the one hand, and its compensation by hypertrophy of the muscle on the other hand, may reach an equilibrium which, as indicated, may last for long periods of time. In such cases an additional factor may upset this equilibrium and lead to heart failure. Such additive factors include an intercurrent infection, the performance of unusually strenuous exercise, damage to the myocardium, and the development of anemia. Since some such events may occur abruptly, it is not unusual to find a patient who has been well compensated for years suddenly develop heart failure.

The *second cause* of cardiac failure is the abrupt development of an increased work load without sufficient time for the heart to adapt itself by compensatory hypertrophy. This may happen in patients whose heart valve is suddenly destroyed from an injury or severe infection, or who abruptly develop hypertension within either of the two circuits. The *third cause* of cardiac failure is damage to heart muscle, which becomes incapable of properly handling the normal circulatory load. Such damage to the heart occurs with destruction of portions of the heart muscle from diseases of the coronary circulation and with various inflammatory and metabolic involvements of the myocardium, to be discussed in chapters 9 and 14.

The seriousness of the condition of a patient in heart failure depends mostly on two factors: the severity of the derangement of the circulatory functions and the speed of development of heart failure. Acute failure of the heart is, as a general rule, more serious than its chronic form, since so much depends upon the capability of the various body functions to adapt themselves to a "low-budget" circulation; such adaptation requires time. Thus, acute pulmonary edema due to sudden left ventricular failure may be fatal because the lungs cannot cope, unprepared, with the excess fluid and the high pressure. However, these same physiological derangements developing less abruptly could easily be tolerated. Nonfatal, acute heart failure produces severe symptoms which usually bring the physician early, permitting effective treatment. On the other hand, gradual onset of chronic heart failure may be so inconspicuous, especially in patients who customarily engage in limited physical activities, that the patient may be unaware of the presence of serious heart disease. Such patients may misinterpret their symptoms as "colds," try self-treatment, and not see the physician until advanced stages of heart failure are present. We once saw a patient who first sought medical care only after 130 pounds of excess fluid had accumulated in his body!

The *diagnosis* of heart failure is easy in its fully developed stage. However, early recognition of heart failure, particularly when the patient's disability is not very pronounced, as sometimes occurs, may present considerable difficulties for the physician. The diagnosis sometimes may have to rely on minor or indirect clues, such as changes in heart sounds, "congestion" shown in the chest X ray, and certain laboratory tests. It should be emphasized once more that the electrocardiogram is totally useless as an aid in distinguishing the state of compensation from heart failure.

Treatment of heart failure has three objectives:

1) Reduction of cardiac overload. Theoretically all processes leading to heart failure—hypertrophy, dilatation, and failure—are reversible. To what extent this is possible in conditions with chronic long-standing overload is not known. If the increased work load is caused by mechanical, surgically correctable defects, reversal of failure may take place along with reduction of heart size. In such cases one can think in terms of complete cure. However, this is rare. More often surgical or medical treatment may be capable of partly relieving the overload, and this, in turn, may restore the state of compensation. In conditions in which the original cause of the overload cannot be eliminated or reduced, the removal of some secondary forms of overloading of the circulation may benefit the patient. Among possible steps to be taken are: treatment of intercurrent infections, reduction of excess body weight, correction of anemia, and elimination of exercise. Periods of "complete bed rest" (see chap. 5) seldom are prescribed for chronic heart failure, but if they are they fall into the category of reduction of overload.

2) Improvement of cardiac performance by drugs. The principal agent for this purpose is digitalis, the action of which has been discussed in chapter 5. Digitalis is particularly effective when heart failure is associated with a disturbance of cardiac rhythm, wherein *both* actions of this drug contribute to the beneficial effect upon the circulation. Digitalis may strengthen myocardial contraction sufficiently to improve cardiac performance and restore compensation even if the overload is left unchanged.

In addition to digitalis there are other cardiac "tonics" capable of strengthening cardiac contraction and improving performance. Some such drugs have found application in short-term emergency treatment.

3) Elimination of excess salt and water. This approach to the problem has already been discussed. It has been pointed out that such an effect can be brought about by diuretic drugs, by salt restriction in the diet, or by a combination of both. The use of diuretic drugs may exert the most spectacular effect upon patients with heart failure: a single injection of a diuretic may lead to large-scale elimination of excess fluids, shown by a weight loss of as much as 15 pounds. In such cases, within hours after the injection, relief of symptoms occurs and striking improvement in the patient's condition may become apparent.

The fate of patients in heart failure varies considerably. The outcome is related to the basic cause of the disorder, the immediate cause of failure, and the response to treatment. As a rule, patients improve somewhat, especially in their first bout of failure. In some cases, a state of compensation can be restored and the patients maintained in it for long periods of time. In others, failure may merely be kept in abeyance by continuous therapy, although even in such cases patients may remain free from major symptoms. The possibility of a complete "cure" in rare instances has already been mentioned. In some patients treatment is ineffective and gradual deterioration may occur, particularly when active damage to the heart muscle persists or progresses. The management and supervision of the patient in heart failure, or recovering from it, may present a real challenge to the physician, for under his guidance, with good cooperation from the patient, an individual with even serious heart damage may still maintain freedom from symptoms and engage in a useful, reasonably active life.

7

Alterations of the Rhythm of the Heart

The action of the heart hinges upon its rhythmic contractions, and consequently the most important feature of heart function—the sine qua non of life—is the rhythmic formation and propagation of the electric impulses which stimulate the heart muscle to its contraction. In chapter 3 the delicate regulating mechanisms and the system of checks and balances involved in the formation and the conduction of impulses were presented. This chapter deals with what happens if the system goes out of order, if its mechanisms are impaired. Considering the importance of heart rhythm, it is fortunate that most disturbances of the sequence of beats are of relatively minor importance to the function of the heart, thanks to the intricate safeguards against serious disruptions of heart rhythm. However, if the heart is already weakened by disease, then such disturbances may significantly impair circulatory functions. Furthermore, on rare occasions the system of safeguards may fail and the resulting total or near-total breakdown of the heart rhythm may have disastrous consequences.

GENERAL DEFINITIONS AND NORMAL VARIATIONS

Normal individuals have a regular sequence of heart action with a rate of about 70 beats per minute when resting. The process of impulse formation and its conduction from the pacemaker to the ventricles has been described in chapter 3. The regularity of the heartbeat, its rate, and the origin and spread of impulses, all can undergo deviations from the norm. The over-all term covering these abnormalities, regardless of their origin or significance, is *arrhythmia*—disturbance of heart rhythm. This term is used in its widest sense, even if the regular sequence of beats is not disturbed as a result of this process.

The normal heartbeat is carefully regulated. At rest the rate is within relatively narrow limits between 60 and 80 beats per minute in adults; the normal rate in children is higher. During excitement and exercise the heart rate rises. The highest rate attained during strenuous exercise is between 160 and 200. The normal pacemaker, as stated, is located in the sinoatrial node (S-A note). The rhythm, under normal circumstances, is called sinoatrial rhythm, or, for short, *sinus rhythm*. It is customary to limit this term, sinus rhythm, to moderate rates between the ranges of 60 to 100. When the heart rate exceeds 100 beats per minute it is referred to as "rapid rate" or *tachycardia,* regardless of whether this represents a normal phenomenon (such as exercise) or is abnormal. Conversely, a rate below 60 beats per minute becomes "slow rate" or *bradycardia.* Slow or rapid rate may still originate in the normal pacemaker, then called *sinus bradycardia* and *sinus tachycardia,* or may be a manifestation of an abnormal rhythm. Abnormal ranges of impulse formation in the S-A node, when not caused by such factors as exercise and excitement, are usually related to signals from the nervous system and are more often manifestations of disturbances outside the heart than of heart disease. For example, tachycardia occurs with fever or shock; bradycardia may develop during certain forms of faints or with nausea.

The normal rhythm of the heartbeat is almost perfectly regular. There are times, however, when an irregularity of the rhythm is entirely due to a variation of the sequence of firing in the S-A node. Such irregularities are called *sinus arrhythmia* and are usually related to the effects of the respiration, such as slight slowing of the rate during inspiration, and speeding during expiration. This is not considered abnormal, but merely a variant of the norm. It is observed especially frequently in children.

The significance of these normal variants—sinus bradycardia, sinus tachycardia, and sinus arrhythmia—lies in the realization that they do not represent real disturbances of the heartbeat. The identification of their normal mechanism can be made with the aid of the electrocardiogram. They should be contrasted and separated from real disturbances of cardiac rhythm, which will be discussed below. Such disturbances are customarily divided into abnormalities of impulse formation and abnormalities of impulse conduction.

DISORDERS OF IMPULSE FORMATION

The sinoatrial node, as the primary pacemaker, has the strongest and most reliable rhythmic properties of impulse formation. It has been stated, however, that other parts of the conducting system also have such properties, even though less pronounced. If for any reason the heart is activated from an impulse originating *outside* the S-A node, the abnormal origin of the beat is indicated by the use of the term *ectopic*. Ectopic impulses or rhythms may originate at any point along the pathway of the impulse through the heart. The three principal points of abnormal impulse formation (*ectopic focus*) are: (*a*) the atrium, (*b*) the A-V node, and (*c*) the conducting system within the ventricles. Consequently ectopic foci are referred to as *atrial, nodal,* and *ventricular.* Each focus may fire single beats or groups of beats, or may take over the entire job of impulse formation, becoming an ectopic pacemaker.

There are two reasons why an ectopic focus may fire impulses:

1) When the ectopic focus become unduly active (*irritable focus*), stronger than the S-A pacemaker.

2) When impulses from above fail to come, either because of failure of the S-A pacemaker or blockage of the pathway, in which case the ectopic focus exercises its role as emergency pacemaker.

In spite of the fact that there are three areas for the formation of abnormal impulses (see above), it is customary to combine the atrial and nodal foci together and to discuss arrhythmias in terms of two principal forms of ectopic rhythms: (*a*) supraventricular (atrial or nodal), and (*b*) ventricular.

ECTOPIC BEATS

Single beats originating in an ectopic focus are called *ectopic beats* or *extrasystoles*. These beats are usually caused by temporary irritability of such a focus and appear prematurely, *before* the anticipated next beat from the S-A node. These beats are therefore also referred to as *premature beats*. They almost always cause cancellation of the next beat after them, since the ventricles are nonresponsive at the time the normal impulse reaches them. This is shown in figure 23, in which an ectopic beat, 5, occurs after beat 4. The canceled normal beat 5 is shown by the dotted line. It is seen that after an ectopic beat there is a longer interval before the next beat; this is called *compensatory pause*. It is noteworthy that the interval between beats 4 and 6 is the same as between any other three beats. Ectopic beats originating from any focus occur frequently in normal individuals and usually carry no special significance except occasionally, as a nuisance, when more sensitive individuals experience an unpleasant "void"

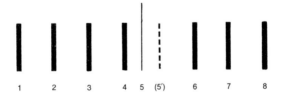

FIGURE 23. *Diagram showing the sequence of heartbeats with the rhythm disrupted by a premature (ectopic) beat. The premature beat is shown by a thinner line (5). It cancels out the next normal beat (shown by the dotted line, 5′); hence there is a longer, "compensatory" pause following the premature beat.*

sensation due to the longer pause between beats (*skipped beat*).

While simple ectopic, premature beats are seldom of significance, the presence of repetitive ectopic beats may be of some importance; such irritability of a focus can occur in healthy individuals as well as those with heart disease. Repeated ectopic beats may occur at haphazard intervals, or may show a specific relationship to beats originating in the S-A node. Among the latter is the important form of arrhythmia, *bigeminal rhythm,* in which each beat from the S-A node is followed by an ectopic beat.

As a general rule ectopic beats from the *atrium* or the A-V node, even when occurring repetitively, are of little significance. Such beats originating in the *ventricle* also may be innocent, though under some circumstances they may be of significance, even of grave consequence. For example, bigeminal rhythm due to ventricular ectopic beats may represent a toxic effect of digitalis, a precursor of more serious, fatal arrhythmias which might develop if the drug is not stopped.

TACHYCARDIAS

Ectopic tachycardias represent a common abnormality of cardiac rhythm consisting of a rapid and regular heartbeat which may originate in an overactive atrial or nodal (*supraventricular*) focus or from a ventricular focus. Usually they represent a temporary disturbance of rhythm with sudden onset and sudden termination, although occasionally a chronic, semipermanent form of ectopic tachycardia may develop. Circumscribed attacks are called *paroxysms,* and are identified as *paroxysmal atrial tachycardias, paroxysmal nodal tachycardias* (*supraventricular*), or *paroxysmal ventricular tachycardias.* Paroxysmal tachycardias vary in rate and duration; some may have rates only slightly higher than normal rhythm, say, 120 beats per minute. At times extremely rapid tachycardias occur, with rates in excess of 200 beats per minute. They may last minutes, hours, or even days.

Supraventricular tachycardias are, as mentioned, less significant than ventricular tachycardias. They occur at least as often, or more often, in individuals without heart disease as they do in cardiac patients. They are usually considered innocent disturbances of heart rhythm; shorter attacks may not need any treatment, and longer ones can usually be brought under control by appropriate medication. Ventricular tachycardias, on the other hand, are considered highly significant, even grave, events in the course of heart disease. Though occasionally occurring without heart disease, ventricular tachycardias develop mostly in seriously ill patients and require active and prompt treatment.

FLUTTER AND FIBRILLATION

These disorders represent the most serious forms of disturbance of impulse formation: partial disorganization of the action (flutter) or total disorganization of heart action (fibrillation). Such disorders may affect either the atria or the ventricles. Atrial flutter or fibrillation represents a relatively common condition which may or may not significantly affect the circulatory functions; ventricular flutter and fibrillation is immediately fatal unless successfully treated at once. This difference is self-evident: loss of atrial function due to disorganization may not disrupt cardiac performance; disorganization of ventricular action is tantamount to complete stoppage of the circulation, for pumping action becomes nil.

Atrial flutter represents rapid, semiorganized action of the atria at an average rate of 300 atrial beats per minute. Such impulses, transmitted through the heart's conducting system, find the ventricles incapable of responding so rapidly; as a rule every other beat arrives during a nonresponsive stage of the ventricles, and hence ventricular contractions occur at one-half the atrial rate. Atrial action usually occurs at perfectly regular intervals, and hence the ventricles beat at regular intervals 150 times per minute. Sometimes, particularly in response to drugs, conduction from the atria is further impaired; the ventricles then respond to every third or fourth atrial impulse and show a rate of 100 or 75 beats per minute. The origin of atrial flutter is not entirely understood. The most widely accepted theory postulates an abnormal state of the atria during which a continuous impulse travels around the two atria (*circus movement*) at a rate of about 300 beats per minute, providing uninterrupted electrical activity and resulting in a fluttering motion of these chambers. The alternate theory suggests a very rapidly discharging ectopic atrial focus—a variant of rapid atrial tachycardia.

Atrial fibrillation is one of the commonest forms of arrhythmia. It occurs most commonly in specific types of heart disease, such as in disorders of the mitral valve, but occasionally is found in individuals who have no detectable cardiac disease. In atrial fibrillation the electrical activity is even faster than in atrial flutter and leads to a total mechanical disintegration of atrial function, so that direct observation of fibrillating atria reveals merely uncoordinated twitching of the atrial musculature. Atrial fibrillation has many features similar to atrial flutter: in both, the ventricles can only respond to a small number of atrial stimuli; both may occur in the same individual at different times; in both the origin is thought to be related to a continuous atrial impulse wave (circus movement; see above). In spite of the lack of coordination in atrial fibrillation a certain number of atrial impulses can be demonstrated by electrocardiography, their number being between 400 and 500 per minute. These impulses are unequal in their capability to stimulate the ventricles: some are stronger than others. The ventricles, able to respond to no more than 200 impulses per minute, are stimulated by the stronger impulses which appear at irregular intervals, and consequently the rhythm of the ventricles is totally irregular. The sensitivity of ventricular responses to atrial fibrillatory twitchings can be regulated by drugs, particularly by digitalis (see chap. 5). In a patient who develops atrial fibrillation and has not been treated, ventricular rate usually varies between 150 and 180 beats per minute; after administration of digitalis the rate can be slowed to 100, 75, or even 50 beats per minute, depending upon the dose of this drug.

Ventricular flutter and fibrillation represent disorganization of the action of ventricular musculature by a mechanism similar to the equivalent atrial arrhythmias. As mentioned, these ventricular arrhythmias stop pumping action of the heart and produce *cardiac arrest,* which is tantamount to death unless resuscitation is instituted within four minutes or less (critical time limits for survival of the brain without circulation). Except on the rare occasions in which a spontaneously terminating paroxysm of ventricular flutter or fibrillation lasting less than one minute occurs, these arrhythmias represent the most dreaded complications of heart disease; they are the commonest mechanism of sudden death in patients with heart disease. Such an event may occur in any form of serious heart disease, but is particularly common in diseases of the coronary circulation. Occasionally ventricular fibrillation may develop as a result of toxic drug action. The only effective measures for ventricular flutter and fibrillation are their prevention by effective treatment in response to certain danger signs. In some conditions associated with temporary proneness to these arrhythmias, special monitoring devices may place the patient within reach of immediate help and save his life.

DISORDERS OF CARDIAC CONDUCTION

The pathway of impulses from the pacemaker to the ventricular wall has been described in chapter 3 and illustrated in figure 11. The process of conduction of impulses can be disturbed in three ways:

1) By a delay at a given point.
2) By its total interruption somewhere along the course.
3) By nonresponsiveness of some part of the pathway.

Delay of conduction occurs usually between the atria and ventricles, presumably by slowing the transit of the impulses through the A-V node. Such a delay is shown in the electrocardiogram by the fact that the interval between the P-wave and the QRS-complex is prolonged beyond the normal time of 0.2 second. This phenomenon is called *first-degree heart block* (fig. 24*b*). This disturbance may appear in the course of some acute illnesses with involvement of the heart and may be the result of drug action. First-degree heart block does not disturb the rhythm or the rate

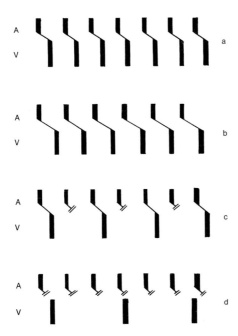

FIGURE 24. *Diagram showing the sequence of beats under normal conditions and in various forms of heart block. The upper bar (A) represents atrial contraction; the lower bar (V), ventricular contraction. The oblique line joining the two bars is the atrioventricular conduction.*

a. Normal conduction.

b. First-degree heart block, showing a delayed atrioventricular conduction, hence longer interval between contraction of the atria and the ventricles.

c. Second-degree heart block, showing every other beat blocked and prevented from reaching the ventricle. The ventricular rate is one-half that of the atria.

d. Complete heart block. All communication between the atria and the ventricles is interrupted. Consequently, the atria and the ventricles beat independently of each other, the ventricular rate usually being much slower than the atrial rate.

of the heart; it is primarily detected by the electrocardiograph; its importance lies in the demonstration that the condition system is imperfect; it may precede more serious forms of conduction disturbances.

A higher degree of impairment of conduction between the atria and the ventricles manifests itself as *second-degree heart block,* a condition in which a certain number of impulses from the atria never reach the ventricle (fig. 24*c*). Thus, one out of every two, three, four or more impulses from the atria is lost, producing *dropped beats.* The result may be an irregular heart action (if dropped beats occur every third beat or more), or a regular rhythm (if every other beat is dropped—*two to one heart block*).

The next step in the process of disturbed atrioventricular conduction is its total interruption, *third-degree heart block,* also called *complete heart block.* Here a completely independent action of the atria and ventricles takes place: the atria contract as a result of the normal S-A mechanism; the ventricles contract as a result of a "ventricular" pacemaker with its slow rhythm (see chap. 3), unrelated to the atrial activity (fig. 24*d*). In complete heart block the atria usually maintain the normal heart rate of 70 beats per minute; the ventricles beat only 30 to 40 times per minute. This unusually slow ventricular rate imposes obvious problems upon the maintenance of the circulation. In an otherwise well-performing heart the circulation can be maintained reasonably well, especially if activities are restricted; in the presence of serious heart disease such a low rate may precipitate heart failure. However, the principal danger of complete heart block lies in the fact that the ventricular pacemaker constitutes the "last line of defense": its failure leaves the heart without any impulses—without contraction. Such failure of the ventricular pacemaker occurs occasionally in complete heart block for short periods of time (less than two minutes); such an event manifests itself in loss of consciousness and is known as *cardiac syncope* or *Stokes–Adams attack.* The dangerous nature of such attacks is self-evident: the life of the patient depends upon the short duration of such failure, for extension beyond the critical four minutes would be fatal.

The three degrees of heart block discussed above may be temporary or permanent. Permanency implies complete, organic destruction of the given part of the conduction pathway; temporary heart block may be due to acute, reversible illnesses, to the action of drugs, or to nervous influences.

If the interruption of pathways of conduction occurs in the section below the division of the bundle of His into two branches, the impulse then reaches the ventricle through the healthy bundle, so that the rhythm of the heart is not disturbed. However, if one of the ventricles fails to receive the impulses directly from the conduction pathways and is activated via a detour to the other ventricle, the second ventricle contracts with a slight delay—a fact not necessarily affecting the function of the heart, but causing gross distortion of the electrocardiogram. This type of conduction defect is called bundle-branch block (right or left, depending on which bundle is damaged). Bundle-branch block is a common disorder in some forms of heart disease, particularly in diseases of the coronary arteries.

Disturbances of the conduction system due to nonresponsiveness of the conducting tissues has already been touched upon in connection with atrial flutter and fibrillation, in which not all rapid impulses can reach the ventricles because of such a mechanism. Other conditions in this category include a rare disorder named *atrioventricular dissociation,* in which the A-V node fires at an abnormally high speed, faster than the S-A node, and therefore takes priority in activating the ventricles. Nonresponsiveness of conducting pathways may separate these impulses from the atria, which obey the normal S-A node stimulation. This situation resembles complete heart block in that the atria and the ventricles beat independently from each other, although here, in contrast to complete heart block, atrial rate is *slower* than ventricular rate. Such conditions are almost always temporary, usually of short duration, and often reflect influences of factors outside the heart (drugs or disturbance of salt and water metabolism).

SIGNIFICANCE OF ARRHYTHMIAS

The foregoing discussion presented the essential mechanisms of the commoner arrhythmias; it was indicated that arrhythmias, in general, may develop in healthy individuals as well as in those suffering from serious heart disease. Furthermore, it was pointed out that some arrhythmias in no way alter cardiac performance, while others adversely affect heart function. The discussion of the general significance of arrhythmias thus revolves around two principal questions:

1) Do arrhythmias adversely affect cardiac function and cardiac performance?

2) How important are arrhythmias as manifestations of underlying heart disease?

In attempting to answer the first question it is necessary to separate the normal individual from one with cardiac disease. An abnormality of heart action can be recognized by the physician by one of its three manifestations: (*a*) the heartbeat (or the pulse) may be irregular; (*b*) it may be abnormally rapid; or (*c*) it may be abnormally slow. The performance of the heart is not specifically related to the mode of the spread of excitation through it, provided each ventricle contracts properly. However, the pumping action of the heart is related to the blood delivered to it. Inasmuch as the ventricles fill in diastole, the length of the diastole influences their blood content, for a longer diastole permits more blood to enter the ventricles. Thus, a premature beat is always a weaker one than a beat appearing on time; a beat following a premature beat is stronger than an average one because of the longer pause preceding it (see fig. 23). This represents the self-regulatory mechanism which maintains the output of the heart at an even level in spite of irregular heart action. The same mechanism regulates the output in rapid and in slow forms of cardiac action. This mechanism is so perfect that in an otherwise normal heart the rate can vary from 30 to 200 beats per minute without serious consequences; similarly, totally irregular rhythm will have no adverse effect upon the circulation. To be sure, some patients may become aware of an abnormal heart action, and the unaccustomed sensation may sound quite alarming to them. Yet such disturbances do not necessarily constitute heart disease, as they usually have no important effects. On the other hand, such disturbances, consisting of very slow, very rapid, or irregular heart action occurring in individuals with heart disease, may lead to serious consequences, which are, as a rule, more profound the more advanced the disease. This is the result of poorer adaptability and self-regulation of the diseased heart, because some of the reserve powers necessary for adjustment are already overtaxed. Consequently, the onset of a rapid or irregular heart action in patients with compensated heart disease may lead to heart failure. Arrhythmias are particularly dangerous when cardiac function is temporarily impaired by acute diseases of the heart, such as acute myocardial infarction or myocarditis, or during the healing period after heart surgery. During such critical periods, the development of an otherwise well-tolerated arrhythmia may be very serious or even fatal unless eliminated by prompt treatment.

The significance of arrhythmias as a manifestation of underlying heart disease is also quite variable. Disturbances of impulse formation as a rule indicate that there is a focus wthin the heart which is overactive, "irritable." Such irritability need not indicate heart disease; the most complex arrhythmias occur, at times, in individuals without "organic" heart disease. However, arrhythmia *may* be a manifestation of heart disease, and even the mildest form of it justifies a careful search for the presence of heart disease. The irritability may be caused by an acute or chronic disease of the myocardium, for example, acute myocardial infarction or myocarditis, or a severe degree of cardiac hypertrophy; other possible factors include drugs, toxic agents, and disturbances of electrolyte and acid–alkali balance in body fluids. The cardiac drugs, digitalis and quinidine, are particularly common causes of arrhythmia; even small doses of these drugs in particularly sensitive individuals may cause dangerous arrhythmias.

It has been implied earlier in the discussion that, as a rule, atrial arrhythmias are less serious than ventricular arrhythmias. The reason for this is that the sudden disaster of ventricular flutter or fibrillation (cardiac arrest) is caused by irritability of the ventricles. Consequently, all forms of ventricular arrhythmias, even the most innocent ones, may have some remote connotations of serious consequences; furthermore, ventricular arrhythmias are more likely to indicate heart disease than atrial arrhythmias.

While the foregoing discussion emphasizes the fact that a great proportion of arrhythmias due to disturbances of impulse formation are of little significance or consequence, disturbances of conduction are more ominous. Permanent conduction disturbances almost always mean heart disease, so that higher degrees of heart block not only carry the danger of Stokes–Adams attacks but also can be considered as indicative of serious heart disease.

TREATMENT OF ARRHYTHMIAS

The objectives of therapy of arrhythmias are threefold:

1) The termination of continuous arrhythmias and restoration of "sinus" rhythm.
2) The prevention of intermittent or recurrent arrhythmias.
3) The control of too rapid or too slow heart rates.

Treatment of arrhythmias covers a broad range from the use of innocuous drugs and maneuvers to the application of extensive and risky treatments. It is because of this latter category that the physician has to consider carefully indications for treatment, and to ask himself whether the patient is better off treated or untreated.

The termination of continuous arrhythmias includes the treatment of paroxysmal tachycardias, nonparoxysmal tachycardias, flutter, and fibrillation. The urgency of treatment is related to the respective seriousness of these conditions. Paroxysmal supraventricular tachycardias can frequently be stopped by a reflex initiated by the stimulation of the vagus nerve. This can best be done by applying pressure upon the carotid artery at mid-neck, near the angle of the jaw. Almost half such attacks can be stopped instantly by this simple maneuver. Where this maneuver fails, various drugs can be used, some safe, some potentially dangerous. Treatment then becomes a matter of whether immediate termination of an attack is imperative. In patients with heart disease, who tolerate rapid heart rates poorly, more hazardous types of treatment may be justified. In healthy individuals it may sometimes be best to wait for a spontaneous termination of such an attack, rather than take a risk by using certain toxic drugs if safe drugs are unsuccessful.

Ventricular tachycardia is one of the more serious manifestations of ventricular irritability and is always dangerous; active treatment is then indicated, and the taking of risks is justifiable. Choice of treatment often consists of intravenous use of drugs and electric shock therapy.

The treatment of atrial flutter and fibrillation can be approached in two ways: it may be aimed either at the termination of these arrhythmias or at control of heart rate. The former is usually undertaken in individuals without advanced heart disease or in those whose arrhythmia has developed recently. On the other hand, some patients known to be particularly prone to this arrhythmia are first seen when atrial fibrillation has been present for months or years; then the physician usually prefers to control the heart rate.

The recently introduced electric shock therapy of arrhythmias is one of the most satisfactory forms of treatment. Electric shock has been used for some time as a means of stopping ventricular fibrillation—a dire emergency treatment. It has now been demonstrated that a timed discharge of direct-current electricity may be applied to the skin of the chest, and it is capable of stopping abnormal impulses long enough for the normal pacemaker to take over the rhythm. This method has been successfully applied to the treatment of supraventricular and ventricular tachycardias, atrial flutter, and atrial fibrillation. Successful as it is, electric shock carries a slight risk and has to be given, as a rule, under general anesthesia; hence, simpler means of treatment are usually applied first.

The prevention of intermittent and recurrent arrhythmias requires discriminating analysis in each instance. For example, frequent occurrence of ectopic beats may be annoying for the patient, and yet the slight risk of continuous administration of quinidine for its prevention may not be justifiable. Similarly, some healthy individuals suffer from repeated attacks of paroxysmal tachycardias. In many instances the attacks can be prevented by the continuous use of digitalis or quinidine. Yet in individuals who have such attacks rarely, continuous drug administration may be unwarranted, especially since the attacks are often no more than a minor nuisance to the patient.

The control of heart rate in arrhythmias characterized by too rapid or too slow rates has already been touched upon in this discussion. Whenever termination of a rapid arrhythmia is not indicated, the use of digitalis is the preferred method of treatment. On the other hand, in complete heart block associated with very slow heart rates, the physician has some drugs available which can slightly speed up the rate. Where these are inadequate and the slow rate is poorly tolerated, and in patients who are subject to Stokes–Adams attacks, artificial pacemakers are now available. The introduction of such pacemakers constituted one of the major advances in this field. These pacemakers consist of miniature electronic devices capable of discharging rhythmic electric impulses; they are connected with wires to the heart muscle, which responds to this stimulation by contraction. The pacemakers can either be inserted permanently in the wall of the abdomen and their wires carried under the skin directly to the heart, or they can be applied temporarily through tubes similar to cardiac catheters introduced through the veins and advanced inside the heart. Artificial pacemakers either provide additional stimuli to make the heart beat between the rare natural beats, or may take over the rhythm entirely. Their rate can be regulated according to needs. Since this treatment is a surgical procedure and carries a risk, its use has to be carefully weighed.

Part Three

Diseases of the Heart and Circulation

8

How Heart Disease
Is Classified

Every subject needs an orderly method of presentation, and heart disease is no exception. However, here the systematic arrangement presents considerable difficulties, for it is necessary to account for the cause of the disease, its nature, and the disturbance of the function caused by it. This is particularly important, since most heart diseases represent permanent, lifetime afflictions. One individual may so well tolerate a heart condition that he can lead a normal life in spite of it; another person may be totally disabled by the same condition. An ideal classification of heart disease would permit a physician to express his diagnosis of a patient in such a manner that another physician would have a fairly complete image of the problems involved. The means of achieving such a diagnosis and some of the difficulties encountered are presented in this chapter.

Many diseases present well-defined entities which have clear-cut and specific connotations to the physician and layman alike, for example: appendicitis, infectious mononucleosis, peptic ulcer. Such specific disease entities are few among diseases of the heart. In general, heart disease has so many ramifications that the classification of it is difficult. In order to describe accurately the state of a patient with heart disease in terms of a diagnosis, it is usually necessary to account for four of its aspects: (*a*) the cause of the disease (*etiologic diagnosis*); (*b*) the form in which the *structure* of the heart differs from the norm (*anatomic diagnosis*); (*c*) the presence or absence and the form of physiological mechanisms of the heart (*physiologic diagnosis*); and (*d*) the degree of limitation of the patient's activities (*functional classification*). The necessity to include a four-way description of each case of heart disease imposes considerable difficulties upon the orderly presentation of the various diseases of the heart. Thus, this brief chapter is included as an introduction to the various forms of heart disease and will, it is hoped, help to clarify some points and obviate the need for repeating some parts of the discussion.

The *etiology* of heart diseases usually signifies their origin, but that does not always imply that the exact cause of the disease is understood. The majority of cases fall into four groups, which one is tempted to refer to as the "big four" of heart diseases. These are: (*a*) heart disease due to disturbances of the coronary circulation, (*b*) heart disease due to hypertension (high blood pressure), (*c*) rheumatic heart disease, and (*d*) congenital heart disease. In each one of these groups there is a sequel in the form of specific abnormalities in the heart or blood vessels which appears as a characteristic and easily identifiable pattern, and yet in none of them are the cause and the mechanism entirely known. Thus, diseases of the coronary arteries produce well-known "heart attacks" and specific damage to the heart muscle; however, the cause of atherosclerosis is not known. Rheumatic fever attacks valves of the heart in a characteristic manner, but its exact mechanism and cause are not clearly understood. Similarly, the cause of many birth defects is still unknown; only a small fraction of cases of hypertension are related to known mechanisms.

Among other forms of heart disease there are a few in which there is a clear-cut relationship between cause and effect. In this category one can include heart diseases due to trauma (injury), bacterial infection of the heart valves (endocarditis), inflammatory diseases of the myocardium due to virus infection (virus myocarditis), heart diseases caused by thyroid disease, and heart diseases due to nutritional deficiencies.

Anatomic diagnosis is concerned with the structural changes which can be detected by the pathologist at autopsy or by the surgeon at the operating table. It involves changes in the pericardium, myocardium, or endocardium and diseases of the arteries and veins. Anatomic diagnosis is the traditional means of presentation of heart disease and has dominated the field in the past.

Physiologic diagnosis deals with the disturbances of the various functions of the circulatory system. This includes the entire field of arrhythmias (chap. 7); alteration of cardiac function, such as heart failure (chap. 6); and various specific manifestations of heart diseases referred to as *syndromes*.

Functional classification of heart disease constitutes the physician's appraisal of the patient's disability due to cardiac disease. It has been stated that the patient's capacity to perform physical work may be seriously impaired by symptoms caused by heart disease, primarily shortness of breath and chest pain. Functional capacity of the patient is evaluated as a basis for the classification, regardless of which symptoms limit activities, provided they are related to his heart disease.

Some years ago the New York Heart Association developed a simple classification of the functional status of cardiac patients, which is now universally accepted and used. Patients are divided into four classes:

Class I. Patients who have organic heart disease, but can perform all customary activities without significant symptoms.

Class II. Patients who have symptoms when performing ordinary, moderately strenuous activities. They tolerate less than ordinary activities well and are fully comfortable at rest.

Class III. Patients who are restricted by symptoms, so that less than ordinary activities, even minor ones, produce discomfort; they are, however, comfortable at rest.

Class IV. Patients who can perform no physical activities without some discomfort and usually have symptoms at rest as well.

Since this classification is based upon patients' symptoms, a subjective manifestation of disease (see chap. 4), functional classification is usually made from the patient's medical history. The accuracy of this classification is thus contingent upon the capability of the patient to give an accurate account of his symptoms of heart disease. It has been stated in chapter 4 that a reliable history can be obtained from many but not all patients. It is therefore sometimes necessary to reinforce the interview by actual observation of a patient's performance. This can either be done informally by asking the patient to perform simple exercises, or by more quantitative functional tests, such as walking on the treadmill at a specified speed and incline.

It should be apparent to the reader that the functional classification is in some respects related to the problem of cardiac performance: in cases where the determinant of the intolerance of effort is shortness of breath, gradual reduction of activities is associated with the change from compensated heart disease into heart failure. Usually, patients with chronic heart disease who are in Classes I and II are compensated; those in Classes III and IV are in heart failure. There are, however, exceptions to this rule.

Since the functional capability of a patient to perform work often ties in closely with the physician's recommendation as to how much activity he should engage in, a companion classification of activities has been developed which is intended to code the physician's orders concerning the patient's activity. This is the *therapeutic classification:*

Class A. Patients are permitted to undertake unlimited physical effort.

Class B. Patients' only restriction concerns avoidance of severe or competitive effort.

Class C. Patients' ordinary physical activities are moderately restricted and strenuous activities altogether eliminated.

Class D. Patients are permitted to engage only in minor activities.

Class E. Patients are placed on a rest regimen, confined to bed or chair.

These five classes represent the range of medical recommendations referred to in chapter 5. Some such recommendations are permanent; others are temporary and are revised periodically, depending upon the progress of the patients. There is usually a close relationship between the functional and the therapeutic classification: patients in Class I are often placed in Class A; those in Class IV usually rate Class E. However, there are some situations in which it is necessary to restrict the patient more than his symptoms would indicate. Under certain circumstances asymptomatic patients (Class I) are placed on complete rest (Class E). The reasons for this will be mentioned in connection with acute diseases of the heart (chap. 9).

The evolution of the multiphasic classification of heart disease discussed in this chapter has simplified the diagnostic evaluation of patients with diseases of the heart to a considerable extent, and has made a diagnosis more comprehensible and meaningful. However, in the last few years the sharply defined requirements for the modes of classification have begun to blur. The traditional approach to diagnosis consisting of emphasis upon the etiology and structural abnormalities has been replaced in many situations by thinking first in terms of the various physiological disorders that can now be determined by cardiac catheterization techniques. Furthermore, surgical treatment of heart disease has necessitated a regrouping of certain unrelated diseases because of the similiarity of the surgical approach to them. As a consequence of this, the discussion that is to follow will not proceed strictly along the lines of etiology and anatomy of heart disease, as it would were this book written in the mid-1950's.

9

Acute Diseases
of the Heart

The perpetually beating heart may appear to be an organ vulnerable to disease. In reality, its toughness and resilience make it one of the strongest organs in the human body. Nowhere are these features better shown than in acute diseases of the heart, where serious infection or inflammation of the various layers of the heart may temporarily derange its action but where the normal processes of repair and adaptation bring about complete recovery.

Most diseases of the circulatory system are chronic in nature, often permanent. Acute forms of heart disease include episodes in the course of chronic disease (such as myocardial infarction) and a small number of inflammatory diseases of the heart, which are presented in this chapter. These diseases are often characterized by sudden onset, by fever, and by generalized ill-feeling. They may result in death or in complete cure; some can lead to partial recovery or to a permanent and continuous affliction of the heart. The four most important conditions in this category are: rheumatic carditis, bacterial endocarditis, acute myocarditis, and acute pericarditis. They all represent an inflammatory reaction of cardiac tissues, as the suffix *-itis* indicates.

RHEUMATIC FEVER
Rheumatic fever is one of the most important causes of chronic heart disease. It is a disease which shows a wide range of vari-

132

ability, producing an acute illness with well-defined, easily recognized features in some cases, and only minimal, easily overlooked symptoms in others. Though the subject of extensive research for many decades, rheumatic fever has some aspects which are as yet incompletely understood.

Rheumatic fever is not an infectious disease in the ordinary sense; that is, it is not the direct result of the entry of microorganisms (bacteria or viruses) into the body and into the tissues affected by this disease. However, it bears close relationship to the *hemolytic streptococcus,* an organism responsible for many attacks of sore throat, particularly in children. Among the many arguments demonstrating the relationship between rheumatic fever and streptococcal infection, the most convincing ones are as follows: (*a*) acute rheumatic fever is usually preceded by sore throat of streptococcal origin, which occurs as a rule two to four weeks earlier; (*b*) patients suffering from rheumatic fever almost invariably have in their blood antibodies proving recent exposure to hemolytic streptococcus; (*c*) cure of streptococcal infection by penicillin may not prevent the later development of rheumatic fever, but prevention of streptococcal infection protects from rheumatic fever; (*d*) experimental studies succeeded in reproducing in rabbit tissue changes similar to human rheumatic stigmata when streptococci were injected in the animals' skins. Yet, in patients suffering from rheumatic fever, hemolytic streptococci cannot ordinarily be found or cultured from their blood.

Thus, the relationship between the hemolytic streptococcus and rheumatic fever is an *indirect* one. An individual affected by streptococcal sore throat may become sensitized by this germ; when reexposed to it later he may develop an abnormal reaction to it by producing "rheumatic" tissue changes. Rheumatic fever represents a series of abnormal immuno-chemical tissue reactions which fall into the category of "hypersensitivity phenomena" somewhat similar to the serious tissue reactions which occur occasionally after the administration of a serum (serum sickness) or in some forms of drug allergy.

The epidemiology of rheumatic fever is of considerable interest in that there are striking regional differences in its occurrence, which are only in part explained by different climates. In the United States, the New England, North Atlantic, and Rocky Mountain states have the highest incidence of rheumatic fever; the Great Lakes region a slightly lower; and the South and Far West have the lowest incidence. Other factors in the epidemiology of this disease include age prevalence: the susceptibility to rheumatic fever starts at about the age of four, reaches its peak at about ten, and declines sharply after the age of 20. Furthermore, there is a distinct family prevalence of rheumatic fever, in that certain families appear to have high susceptibility to this disease, while others do not. Finally, crowding has an important influence upon the susceptibility to rheumatic fever. This is shown by the fact that it occurs much more frequently in areas with substandard housing. Also, true epidemics of rheumatic fever occur from time to time in army barracks, even though adults have low susceptibility to this disease.

Rheumatic fever involves many tissues and organs of the body. It manifests itself as scattered microscopic areas of accumulation of inflammatory cells invading various tissues. These groups of cells were first described by the German pathologist Aschoff and carry the name of *Aschoff bodies*. The acute manifestations of rheumatic fever are as follows:

1) *Polyarthritis,* nonsimultaneous "migrating" involvement of the larger joints—knees, elbows, ankles, and hips—with periods of painful swelling lasting a few days and then invading other joints.

2) *Pancarditis,* involvement of all three layers of the heart (endocardium, myocardium, and pericardium).

3) *Erythema multiforme,* transient rashes or small nodules under the skin.

4) *Chorea* (St. Vitus' dance), uncoordinated, jerky involuntary movements of the face and extremities.

5) *Pneumonia* and *pleurisy.*

The most typical picture of rheumatic fever is an acute illness involving the joints and the heart. Rheumatic arthritis often is associated with high fever and may last from two to several weeks, although treatment may make the patient comfortable within days. Such typical attacks cause the physician no difficulty in recognizing the illness early. However, rheumatic fever frequently occurs in less typical forms, which consist of only minor joint involvement or in which joints are altogether spared. Then the diagnosis of rheumatic fever may be difficult.

Since rheumatic fever is an acute illness, the tiny Aschoff nodules eventually heal and leave no significant aftereffects. Thus, regardless of how severe the attack of arthritis, the condition of the joint returns to normal; chronic arthritis is virtually unknown as a consequence of rheumatic fever. Similarly, chorea may produce temporary disability by the uncoordinated, jerky, and involuntary movements of the child's extremities, but after weeks or months normal function is restored. Pneumonia, a rare and serious manifestation of rheumatic fever, leaves no after-effects. Along with the other manifestations, the acute phase of rheumatic involvement of the heart is also reversible and heals promptly. However, rheumatic nodules frequently invade the delicate valves of the heart and there may produce permanent damage. Paradoxically, the actual invasion of the heart valves by rheumatic fever produces damage less frequently than the *healing* process: as the nodules heal, the valves become foreshortened, thickened, and may develop faulty function, either by becoming too narrow for the orifice or by becoming incompetent. The treacherous nature of rheumatic fever thus becomes obvious: regardless of how severe or mild the attack may be, it is impossible to predict whether in the future chronic heart disease will or will not develop.

Looking at rheumatic fever from the viewpoint of heart disease, one can thus recognize two stages: (*a*) the stage of *active* disease, and (*b*) the *inactive* stage of valve damage and its consequences upon the heart. The second stage will be covered in a later chapter (chap. 12). The problem of active rheumatic carditis is one of considerable complexity: first, active carditis may persist a long time after the other manifestations or rheumatic fever have disappeared; second, active carditis may occur in the presence of such mild general rheumatic manifestations that the nature of the disease may be overlooked, or the attack may even be missed altogether. Third, the ultimate outcome— the seriousness of permanent damage to the heart—bears no relationship to the severity of the acute manifestations of carditis. It is therefore possible to find patients who have serious rheumatic valve disease but who have no knowledge or recollection of ever having had rheumatic fever. There also are those who have recovered from near-fatal attacks of rheumatic carditis without showing permanent cardiac aftereffects.

The involvement of the heart by rheumatic fever is by far the most serious manifestation of this disease, not only for its immediate effects but also as a seed for future disease of heart valves. Consequently, the detection of cardiac involvement—not always easy—requires careful investigation by the clinician. Rheumatic involvement of the heart is often referred to as *pancarditis,* afflicting all three layers of the heart. The pericardium is affected frequently, but its involvement is of least significance, from both the immediate and long-range standpoint. The invasion of the myocardium by the rheumatic process—rheumatic myocarditis—is the most serious consequence of rheumatic fever: heart failure caused by massive damage to the myocardium accounts for most fatalities occurring during the acute stage of rheumatic fever. Yet, in the great majority of cases, myocarditis heals and leaves no permanent aftereffects. Rheumatic endocarditis consists of the formation of small nodules upon the inner layer of the heart and upon the heart valves. It has already been mentioned that the immediate damage to the valves is less important than the late effects of the healing of the rheumatic process, which produces diseases of heart valves years later.

Thus, the problem of the recognition of rheumatic fever consists of two parts: the detection of the disease, and the decision whether the heart is or is not affected by it. Both parts of the problem may produce great difficulties. Although attacks associated with migrating arthritis and obvious cardiac involvement present a very clear picture, they occur in a minority of cases. More often than not rheumatic fever presents itself as an ill-defined illness associated with only minor aches in the joints ("growing pains"), mild elevation of temperature, undue tiredness, listlessness, and nosebleeds. The physician dealing with children in the age group of highest susceptibility for rheumatic fever (5 to 15 years) must have a high index of suspicion in order to detect such atypical cases of this disease. However, it is equally important to look upon the problem critically in order to prevent overdiagnosis or rheumatic fever and unnecessary immobilization of children in the growing age.

The diagnosis of rheumatic fever in general, and of carditis in particular, is made by a combination of clinical examination and laboratory tests. The clinical examination is particularly difficult in the atypical cases described above; furthermore, carditis may produce virtually no disability and even no symptoms which would attract attention to the patient's heart. Thus, in patients having rheumatic fever or suspected of having it, the physician has to search carefully for cardiac involvement by repeated physical examinations in order to detect new heart murmurs, abnormal sounds or irregularities of heartbeat, and by frequent electrocardiograms and chest X rays which can sometimes demonstrate evidence of heart involvement. The two principal laboratory tests used as aids in the diagnosis of rheumatic fever (regardless of whether the heart is involved) are the determination of *sedimentation rate* and of the *antistreptolysin titer*. Sedimentation rate is a nonspecific test; an abnormal reading merely indicates an abnormal proportion of some constituents of the blood serum, and therefore is found in a great many infections other than rheumatic fever. The technician measures the speed of settling of red blood cells by collecting a blood sample in a long, thin tube and observing the time for the separation of red cells and serum. The antistreptolysin titer reflects the number of antibodies against the principal product of the hemolytic streptococcus. A high titer indicates that an individual has recently come in contact with this germ; however, this test does not discriminate between the individual who has had a streptococcal sore throat without any consequence and one who has developed the abnormal reaction to it, that is, rheumatic fever. Thus, in practical terms, a high antistreptolysin titer means a "strep" infection (usually sore throat) in the recent past, but not necessarily rheumatic fever. Inasmuch as only a very small fraction of those with "strep" throats develop rheumatic fever, a positive antistreptolysin test occurs many times more often in normal individuals than in those with rheumatic fever. This point deserves special emphasis, for there is a widespread misconception that sedimentation rate and antistreptolysin tests are "tests for rheumatic fever" which are either "positive" or "negative." This is obviously incorrect. Such tests merely provide the physician with a background of information which he considers in the light of clinical findings in each case.

Treatment of rheumatic fever presents several problems. As soon as the diagnosis is made it is customary to put the patient to bed. Bed rest is essential as a means of sparing the work of the heart in cases with myocarditis. However, since myocarditis can often be overlooked, it is assumed that every case of rheumatic fever is a potential case of myocarditis during the active phase of the disease. The second problem involves the possibility that live streptococci may still be present (even though rheumatic fever usually develops weeks after the sore throat). A course of penicillin treatment is recommended for that purpose. The third problem involves specific drugs with the property of reducing inflammatory tissue reaction. These include aspirin and other derivatives of salicylic acid, and various cortisone preparations. In milder cases salicylates are used; in more severe, cortisone. These drugs may have a dramatic effect upon the course of rheumatic fever, but it is still a matter of controversy as to whether intensive anti-inflammatory therapy during the active stage of rheumatic fever will ultimately prevent valve damage.

Perhaps the most important approach to the problem of rheumatic fever is the prevention of a recurrence. The principle of preventive treatment of rheumatic fever is based upon the fact that abnormal sensitivity to the hemolytic streptococcus remains permanently in an individual. As a result, once rheumatic fever has developed, the individual is likely to have further attacks, each time he comes in contact with this germ. It is well known that there is a tendency for rheumatic fever to recur; furthermore, it has been demonstrated that individuals with several attacks of rheumatic fever are more likely to end up with damage to heart valves than those who have had only one attack, and that such damage is more likely to be severe after repeated attacks. It is thus assumed that an individual sensitive to the hemolytic streptococcus will be protected from rheumatic fever if he is protected from coming in contact with this germ. For that purpose a continuous penicillin treatment is used, which has indeed demonstrated that recurrences of rheumatic fever can be drastically reduced, if not eliminated, by such preventive therapy. The only deficiency of this approach is the fact that individuals sensitive to the hemolytic streptococcus can only be detected *after* they come down with an attack of rheumatic fever, which could, of course, have damaged the heart already. Fortunately, the over-all problem of rheumatic fever is on a decline for another reason: the widespread use of antibiotics for children makes the streptococcus a much less common cause of sore throat than in the past; thus the whole population is less exposed to it and hence there is less chance for susceptible individuals to develop hypersensitivity.

Summarizing the subject of rheumatic fever, it should be emphasized that acute rheumatic fever is an illness which is thought to be due to an abnormal hypersensitivity to the hemolytic streptococcus. It is estimated that less than one out of fifty individuals who come down with streptococcal infections will develop this abnormal reaction. Rheumatic fever affects the joints, the heart, the skin, the brain, and the lungs in its acute manifestations, but its involvement of the heart may produce, in certain individuals, permanent damage of cardiac valves.

BACTERIAL ENDOCARDITIS

Endocarditis represents an inflammatory disease of the endocardium. Rheumatic endocarditis has been presented in the preceding section; bacterial endocarditis is another form of endocarditis caused by the lodging of bacteria upon the endocardium. It occurs in two forms: *acute* and *subacute*. The difference between the two is not only in the severity and duration of the infection, but also in the circumstances under which it occurs and the type of organism involved in the infection.

Acute endocarditis, as a rule, is an infection which involves the heart secondarily. Generalized infection of the body caused by an organism with high destructive power (*virulent*) may invade the valves of the heart. The most common cause of acute endocarditis is septicemia (blood-borne dissemination of a serious infection) due to pus-producing bacteria, such as occurs as a complication of serious external, internal, or postsurgical infections. Invasion of heart valves by such organisms often leads to their rapid destruction and may produce fatal heart failure because of the sudden development of valvular insufficiency. In most cases acute endocarditis is not strictly a disease of the heart, but rather a serious general infection of the bloodstream in which the heart becomes implicated. Once the heart is involved, treatment is more difficult and sometimes futile as compared with infections which have not invaded the heart valves.

Subacute bacterial endocarditis is, in contrast, a primary infection of the heart itself. Bacterial infection of the endocardium and the heart valves occurs almost exclusively on areas showing previous damage. Thus the prime targets for subacute endocarditis are cases of rheumatic heart disease or congenital heart disease. The infecting organism is usually one which ordinarily has little destructive power; as a matter of fact, otherwise innocent bacteria may, under certain conditions, invade the heart and cause serious infections. The commonest invader of the heart valve is the green streptococcus (*Streptococcus viridans*), so named because of the greenish color of its colonies when cultured in artificial media. In contrast to its kin, the hemolytic streptococcus, which usually causes disease when invading the human body, the green streptococcus appears to be an innocent inhabitant of the normal mouth in man. Such organisms occasionally get into the bloodstream but are usually easily eliminated by the body's defenses. However, these same streptococci may find and attack a "weak spot," a previously damaged heart valve, and lodge there. There the green streptococcus may grow and multiply, forming small nodules, "vegetations" upon the valves. These vegetations deform heart valves but do not produce extensive destruction such as that in acute endocarditis. The effect of bacterial invasion of heart valves is threefold:

1) The patient shows the effects of an infection, the nature of which may not be apparent. This manifests itself by low-grade fever (often slight afternoon rises of temperature), by generalized weakness, fatigability, and by anemia (pallor).

2) Slow and gradual destruction of heart valves seldom causes rapid development of heart failure, but some degree of insufficiency of heart valves usually becomes apparent; the physician can then detect the appearance of murmurs and other signs.

3) The bacteria-produced vegetations upon the heart valves invite the formation of small clots, which can tear themselves loose and produce *emboli* (occlusion of distant arterial vessels due to the propulsion of an unattached clot with the bloodstream). Such emboli vary in size: minute emboli may reach the skin and form small hemorrhages resembling flea bites (*petechiae*); larger ones may produce painful nodules on the sides of the fingers; still larger may have serious consequences by destroying portions of the brain, causing strokes, or by occluding large arteries to the extremities or to abdominal organs. Small emboli are usually well tolerated by various vital organs, with the exception of the kidneys, which may be seriously damaged by them. Large emboli produce serious consequences and may even be fatal.

Thus, subacute bacterial endocarditis involves two factors: previous damage to heart valves and the entry of the streptococcus, or other organism, into the bloodstream. Valve damage usually represents previously known rheumatic or congenital heart disease. Occasionally endocarditis develops in individuals who have no previous knowledge of heart disease. If this occurs, it is assumed that heart disease was present before, but had not been diagnosed, or that it was of such minor nature that even the most careful examination had not detected it.

The mode of entry of the organism into the bloodstream varies. In some cases this mechanism is obvious, in others unapparent. The most consistently found port of entry occurs in connection with dental surgery. It has been shown that, after dental extractions, the streptococci—normal inhabitants of the oral cavity—often enter the bloodstream but are quickly subdued. It is probable that in many individuals with damaged valves such temporary showers of bacteria after dental surgery are of no consequence. However, sometimes in such individuals these organisms gain a foothold on the damaged valve and start serious trouble. In addition to dental surgery, manipulations upon the urinary tract, surgery on pelvic organs, and even minor pus-producing skin infections occasionally initiate attacks of endocarditis.

The two distinct types of endocarditis, acute endocarditis associated with serious septic infections and subacute endocarditis often caused by *Streptococcus viridans,* present fairly typical pictures. There are, however, many atypical cases in both categories which blur the dividing line between them so that some authorities consider them variants of the same disease. Primary infection of a heart which has previously damaged valves can involve more malignant organisms than the streptococcus and produce a rapid and destructive course. Among the organisms producing such a course is the staphylococcus, which has recently become a serious problem in hospital populations. Staphylococcal endocarditis has been one of the more serious complications of cardiac surgery. Damaged heart valves may be invaded by microorganisms of many different varieties, and there is hardly an organism which has not been reported to cause a case of endocarditis. The notable exceptions, however, are the viruses, which do not ordinarily invade the endocardium.

The diagnosis of subacute bacterial endocarditis rests upon the clinical picture of an infection without obvious source in the presence of rheumatic or congenital heart disease. The various consequences of endocarditis referred to above constitute clues to the diagnosis. However, the most important diagnostic point is the isolation of the causative organism in blood cultures. In endocarditis there are virtually always bacteria in the blood-stream which are fed from the vegetations on the valves. A large sample of blood taken from the patient's vein under sterile conditions is placed on the proper medium to enhance growth of bacteria; "blood culture" permits the identification of the micro-organism in at least 80 percent of cases. This not only proves the diagnosis but provides the guide for effective treatment.

Twenty years ago, acute and subacute bacterial endocarditis were almost uniformly fatal with only rare instances of spontaneous cure, representing less than 1 percent of cases. There was no treatment available, and the patients died either from the infection or from heart failure. The great breakthrough occurred in 1943, when the newly discovered penicillin was shown to be able to cure endocarditis due to *Streptococcus viridans*. With the later introduction of other antibiotics, endocarditis changed from 99 percent fatal to 90 percent curable. The small number of incurable cases represent infections with organisms resistant to antibiotic therapy and cases in which heart failure has progressed in spite of the elimination of the offending organism. Unfortunately, the percentage of curable cases of endocarditis has decreased since the mid-1950's and is now estimated to be at 75 or 80 percent. This is due to the fact that atypical, antibiotic-resistant forms of endocarditis are more often seen now than in the past.

Treatment of bacterial endocarditis has two objectives: the total elimination of the infection, and rapid intervention to prevent damage to the valves and embolic phenomena. Proper treatment thus hinges upon early diagnosis and exact knowledge of the offending germ. Occasionally early diagnosis is impossible because the onset is so inconspicuous that the patient may be unaware that there is something wrong with him. Isolation of the bacteria permits the determination of their sensitivity to various antibiotics, thereby providing a guide as to which antibiotic to use and how high the dose should be. Antibiotic therapy is usually continued long after the patient's condition has returned to normal; this may take but a few days. In order to be sure that all bacteria deeply embedded in the valvular vegetations are killed, it is usually necessary to continue antibiotic therapy for three to six weeks.

It is obvious that the ideal way of dealing with the problem of endocarditis is its prevention. Every patient with rheumatic and congenital heart disease is a potential candidate for endocarditis, with odds somewhere between 5 and 10 percent of acquiring this disease sometime in his life. It is therefore essential to caution such individuals to use undue care in dealing with infections, and to protect them by short courses of antibiotics at the time of dental or other forms of surgery. Such precautions may significantly reduce the risk of endocarditis, although the danger can never be completely eliminated unless surgical cure can eliminate the point of low resistance within the heart (as in some congenital lesions, for example).

ACUTE MYOCARDITIS

Myocarditis refers to an inflammatory process within the heart muscle. Acute myocarditis is relatively rare, but constitutes an important form of heart disease, which may be fatal. A special form of acute myocarditis has already been discussed—rheumatic myocarditis. It has been stated that deaths in acute rheumatic fever are usually due to heart failure, which in turn is caused by myocarditis rather than damage to the valves. *Nonrheumatic myocarditis* occurs mostly as a complication of infections, either localized elsewhere in the body or general in nature. In the past, diphtheritic myocarditis was a dreaded complication of diphtheria, often resulting in death or permanent heart damage. However, effective immunization programs have reduced diphtheria to the ranks of a rare disease. Myocarditis (in contrast to endocarditis) occurs more frequently in connection with virus infections than with those caused by bacteria. Common communicable diseases of childhood are occasionally complicated by myocarditis, particularly mumps. Such diseases as viral hepatitis and infectious mononucleosis can be associated with acute myocarditis. Influenza may cause myocarditis, which probably accounts for a fair number of fatalities due to this disease. In tropical countries myocarditis occurs as a complication of the various infestations with tropical parasites. Finally, myocarditis may occur in various forms of septic bloodstream infections, even as a complication of acute endocarditis when bacteria lodge in the heart muscle and produce abscesses of the myocardium.

Myocarditis has no characteristic features which enable the physician to make the diagnosis readily. As a rule, either the patient is unaware of the fact that his heart may be involved or his attention is drawn to the principal disease of which myocarditis is a complication, although occasionally rapid heart rate or irregularities draw attention to the heart. Physical examination of the heart seldom provides any clues in milder cases. Perhaps the two most important diagnostic clues are: changes in the electrocardiogram and X-ray evidence of enlargement of the heart. However, if involvement of the myocardium is more severe, heart failure may develop. The patient would then experience shortness of breath and the physician would detect the usual signs of heart failure.

Acute myocarditis is always considered a serious complication of infectious diseases, and its outcome is never certain. The crucial point determining its significance is the extent to which heart function is impaired by the inflammatory process; the appearance of heart failure is thus an ominous sign. Yet, even if this occurs, complete recovery is possible. Those who survive acute myocarditis as a rule regain full and normal function of the heart; only occasionally acute myocarditis leads to chronic myocarditis and disabling chronic heart disease.

In contrast to endocarditis, there is no known treatment for myocarditis except strict rest during the active stage.

ACUTE PERICARDITIS

Pericarditis, inflammation of the pericardial sac, can be caused by a great variety of conditions. Infectious agents include viruses, tuberculosis, and various bacteria which can invade the pericardium from the vicinity. Pericarditis occurs as a complication of involvement of other parts of the heart; in rheumatic fever or in myocardial infarction. Pericarditis develops as a complication of uremic poisoning, as a consequence of direct injury (stab wounds or shot wounds), and as a result of invasion by tumors.

As a rule pericarditis occurs in two forms: "dry" pericarditis, and pericarditis with effusion (accumulation of fluid between the two layers of the pericardium). Dry pericarditis often causes pain in the middle of the chest and produces a characteristic noise found on auscultation of the heart (pericardial friction rub). Pericarditis with effusion produces enlargement of the heart visible in the X-ray film and sometimes detectable on examination. The most important consequence of pericardial effusion is its possible interference with cardiac function. Ordinarily, fluid in the pericardial sac does not have any effect upon heart function. However, if excess fluid accumulates too rapidly it may significantly compress the heart to a point where not enough blood can enter from the peripheral circulation, thereby producing symptoms imitating right ventricular failure (see above). This is termed *cardiac tamponade*. Pericarditis with effusion can also be diagnosed from characteristic electrocardiographic changes and by certain changes in the arterial and venous pulse.

Except for the occurrence of cardiac tamponade, which is rather unusual in the course of acute pericarditis, pericarditis is of lesser importance than inflammatory disease of the endo-cardium and the myocardium. Two forms of pericarditis are of special importance: primary pericarditis, of unknown origin (often referred to as *benign idiopathic pericarditis*), and tuber-culous pericarditis. The former occurs often in younger indi-viduals and is associated with chest pain and changes in the electrocardiogram. This may be difficult to distinguish from the infinitely more serious coronary occlusion with myocardial in-farction. Tuberculous pericarditis is important, since it is the only form of pericarditis in which the acute stage may proceed into a chronic form of pericarditis, to be discussed later (*con-strictive pericarditis*).

A special form of pericarditis "allergic" in nature is that re-lated to general hypersensitivity. The membranes lining the cavities of the chest, both the pericardium and the pleura, readily become involved in tissue reaction in various allergic processes. This occurs in some generalized states related to hypersensitivity; it may also follow heart operations as part of the *postcardiotomy syndrome* (a relatively common, transient complication occur-ring a few weeks after heart operations, characterized by chest pain, fever, pericarditis, and pleurisy).

The diagnosis of pericarditis is made on the basis of the vari-ous symptoms, signs, and laboratory findings presented above. In special cases samples of pericardial fluid have to be obtained by needle tap. This is indicated when there is a suspicion of tuberculosis or of pus in the pericardium, or when a cancerous nature of pericardial effusion is deemed possible. In some such cases it may even be necessary to incise the chest in order to obtain biopsy material for more detailed examination.

Treatment of pericarditis is seldom necessary, except for bed rest and the use of drugs to control symptoms. However, if cardiac tamponade occurs and becomes progressively worse, then *pericardiocentesis* (removal of pericardial fluid by needle puncture) may become necessary. This is seldom called for in ordinary medical cases; it is of more importance in cases of in-jury to the heart when the pericardium is filled with blood rather than pericardial fluid. In tuberculous pericarditis drugs for control of tuberculosis are, of course, used. In allergic forms of pericarditis it is occasionally necessary to use cortisone derivatives, but only in unusually severe cases, which are rare.

10

Atherosclerosis and Coronary Disease

Atherosclerosis is generally considered one of the most important health problems—perhaps the number one problem—in affluent populations. As a cause of the commonest form of heart attacks and of strokes, atherosclerosis is responsible for untold cases of disability and death. When the spectacular advances of the last three decades all but eliminated most serious infectious diseases, the medical world began shifting its major interest to "degenerative" diseases—diseases of normal wear and tear. It became obvious that atherosclerosis—a disease of human arteries—does not strictly represent the gradual deterioration with age, but a selective process affecting some individuals, some nations, and some races, but not others. With this premise a world-wide search is now under way to determine the cause of atherosclerosis and the factors involved in its development. The crucial questions, as yet unanswered, are: Is there any means of preventing or postponing atherosclerosis? Is there any factor in the mode of living of the affluent society which makes its population more susceptible to this disease than primitive people are? This chapter contains a statement of the problems and a brief discussion of the difficulties encountered in finding the answers. It also describes the effect of atherosclerosis upon the heart—the interference with the blood supply to the heart itself—coronary disease. Other manifestations of atherosclerosis will be presented in chapter 16.

ATHEROSCLEROSIS

Arteriosclerosis, "hardening of the arteries," is the over-all degenerative process, progressive with age, which produces alterations in the walls of the arteries and results in their increased firmness and tortuosity. This term includes all degenerative changes in the arterial wall, such as the replacement of the elastic tissue in the middle layer of the arterial wall (*media*) by calcium—*mediosclerosis*—and the degenerative process affecting the inner layer (*intima*) of the arterial wall with the appearance of cushion-like "plaques" and the formation of thrombi. This last process is termed *atherosclerosis,* which is the major problem in the field of cardiovascular diseases. The reason for this is quite clear. The arteries serve as the pipelines of communication and can perform well even if their elasticity is altered and their wall thickened. However, a disease process afflicting the inner layer of the arterial wall invariably leads to the formation of overgrowths and clots which narrow, or even occlude, the pipelines, resulting in serious disturbances of the circulation to vital organs. Among the various sites of occlusive diseases of the arteries, the most important is the heart itself. The three coronary arteries supplying blood to the heart are particularly vulnerable to disturbances of the circulation produced by atherosclerosis and have the most serious consequences on health and life. As a result of this, coronary disease has become accepted by those concerned with investigation of atherosclerosis as an index of the atherosclerotic process. For this reason it was felt that the general process of atherosclerosis should be dicussed in connection with coronary disease rather than with diseases of the arteries. However, noncoronary aspects of atherosclerosis will be deferred to a later chapter (chap. 16).

Atherosclerosis is one of the most urgent problems facing medicine today. With the gradual conquest of many other diseases, atherosclerosis stands as a giant against which the medical profession is helpless. Needless to say, the investigations into the nature, causes, treatment, and prevention of atherosclerosis are vast indeed, and involve research at all levels, from chemical studies in the test tube to epidemiological surveys of entire nations. The great volume of information now available permits certain suggestions and trends, but no major breakthroughs have as yet been made.

While the nature of atherosclerosis is not entirely clear, it is generally accepted that it does not represent the direct effect of aging, in the sense of wear and tear on the arteries. It is a specific disease of the arteries, the extent of which varies from individual to individual and the occurrence of which shows a wide range in different nations and races. The actual lesion in the arterial wall consists at first of yellow spots and streaks which develop in the inner lining of the arteries. Such lesions do not interfere with blood flow and are of no significance. Later the progression of this process leads to the development of *plaques,* white, irregular outgrowths from the wall of the artery, which project into the artery and may interfere with blood flow through it. Still later, such plaques may undergo degeneration and develop into ulcers, may show calcium deposits, and are often covered with clots (*thrombi*). These changes provide increasing obstacles to blood flow through the arteries and frequently close these vessels completely by a thrombus filling an entire segment of such an artery.

The causes of these changes in the arteries are not clear. The essential parts of the process, the yellow spots and streaks, are deposits of various fatty substances. Later changes involve fibrous tissue, the nonspecific substance produced by the body in the various processes of healing (scars, etc.), and thrombi. The two major theories concern themselves with whether atherosclerosis is primarily a disturbance of fat metabolism or a disturbance postulating intravascular blood clotting. Both theories have impressive arguments in their favor and both are probably in part correct. It is best to assume that atherosclerosis is caused by an interplay of several factors, of which fat deposition and clot formation are the major ones.

Perhaps the most remarkable fact about atherosclerosis is the extreme variability of its occurrence. On the one hand, it constitutes the leading cause of death in highly civilized countries; on the other hand, it is virtually unknown in some primitive civilizations. The obvious question is, is atherosclerosis preventable? Can we eliminate some factors in our mode of living to protect ourselves against its occurrence, or are we at the mercy of racial differences and heredity? The attempts to answer these fascinating questions occupy the minds of many prominent investigators the world over. In approaching them it is necessary to compare individuals, groups of individuals, and whole nations that have a high incidence of atherosclerosis with those showing a low incidence of it. Many factors have to be included in such an analysis. Some will be discussed briefly.

FAT METABOLISM AND ATHEROSCLEROSIS

Here one has to include: (*a*) fat content in the diet, and (*b*) fat metabolism as shown by the level of fatty substances in the blood. The differences between dietary habits of individuals, regions, and nations provided one of the earlier approaches to the problem. It is clear, by and large, that severe atherosclerosis occurs preferentially in groups of individuals whose diets are rich in fat, particularly of the animal variety. Conversely, inhabitants of regions where atherosclerosis is uncommon usually indulge in diets very low in animal fat.

Fatty substances contained in the human blood include neutral fat and fatty acids, cholesterol and cholesterol esters, and lipoproteins. Each of these components of the human plasma has been considered an important index of the severity of atherosclerosis, although in none can this relationship be considered proven. The undisputable fact is that individuals—and nations—who show low levels of fatty substances in the blood also show low incidence of atherosclerosis; those with high fat content preferentially develop atherosclerosis. The simplest and most widely known and applicable measurement is that of blood cholesterol. The level of blood cholesterol in the average American varies from 180 to 280 mgm. per 100 cc. Some nations with low incidence of atherosclerosis have average cholesterol levels of less than 150 mgm. Individuals with elevated blood cholesterol between 300 and 500 mgm. have an incidence of atherosclerotic heart attacks many times that of the general population. Thus with this information it becomes obvious that a determination of an individual's serum cholesterol may be of some predictive value as to his chances of having heart attacks. This is true only to the extent that the predictive value of a test applies to a statistical probability, which may be of little help in an individual case. For example, if in a certain age group the probability of a "coronary" is 1 in 50, high cholesterol level may change this figure to 1 in 20, or even 1 in 10. However, an individual with high blood cholesterol will still have between 90 or 95 percent probability that he will *not* have a heart attack.

Out of the large body of data concerned with the relationship between atherosclerosis and fat metabolism an attractive theory has evolved. High content of fat (particularly animal fat) in the daily diet produces an overabundance of fatty substances in the blood (shown by a high level of serum cholesterol or other fatty substances) and leads to their deposition in the arterial wall, producing atherosclerosis. Reduction of the fat content in the diet will lower blood fats and prevent atherosclerosis or stop its progression. This theory, with all its plausibility, grossly over-simplifies the problem. The critics point out that it is statistically unsound to single out one factor (fat) in comparing two populations which differ from each other by a large number of factors.

HEREDITY

Strong hereditary factors play an undisputable part in atherosclerosis. Certain families show a high incidence of atherosclerosis and its consequences early in life, regardless of environmental circumstances. Other families seem to be almost immune to this disorder. These tendencies are in part reflected by their serum levels of fatty substances, suggesting an inherited mode of metabolizing fats, but are also related to other, as yet unknown, factors.

HORMONAL INFLUENCES

Some disturbances of glandular function are known to have important influences upon the development of atherosclerosis:

increased activity of the thyroid gland is usually associated with a low level of serum cholesterol and lowered incidence of atherosclerotic complications. In diabetics the cholesterol level is usually elevated, and early atherosclerosis is very common. Ovarian hormones (estrogens) appear to have a protective action against the development of atherosclerosis. This is the basis for the well-known fact that women before menopause have a very much lower degree of atherosclerosis, but after the cessation of ovarian function are just as prone to heart attacks as men.

HIGH BLOOD PRESSURE

Hypertension is one of the most powerful factors known to accelerate the formation of atherosclerosis.

EMOTIONAL STRESS

The effect of stress upon the incidence of atherosclerosis is a subject of considerable discussion in the medical literature. There seems to be some evidence that individuals living under constant stress and tension are subject to more frequent heart attacks than those with well-regulated lives. Some individuals with personality patterns compelling them to competitive drives are thought to have increased probability of heart attacks. Enthusiastic proponents of this relationship suggest stress as one of the principal factors, perhaps the most important single factor, determining the development of atherosclerosis. Other investigators accept stress merely as one of the many factors playing a part in the atherosclerotic process. One reason for this controversy is the difficulty of measuring stress in meaningful terms, in the same way that fatty substances can be measured. Since stress can at best be only roughly estimated, the relationship between atherosclerosis and stress can be expressed only in the most general terms.

OBESITY

Statistical studies demonstrate convincingly that the obese individual is an increased risk in many respects. The incidence of heart disease in general is said to be at least 50 percent higher in overweight individuals than in those with normal weight, as measured by standard mortality statistics. However, specific information linking obesity with acceleration of the atherosclerotic process is not available to the point of being expressed in statistical terms. Obesity adversely affects the function of many organs in the body, including overloading of the circulation, and is likely to be an undesirable factor in a cardiac patient.

TOBACCO

Studies concerned with the effect of smoking upon deaths from heart attacks have demonstrated a significantly higher rate in smokers than in nonsmokers. Such statistics can be considered indirect evidence suggesting that cigarette smoking accelerates atherosclerosis.

EXERCISE

The effect of exercise upon the development of atherosclerosis in general and upon the incidence of heart attacks in particular is subject to the same difficulties of interpretation and control as have been mentioned in connection with other factors. In general it appears that moderate activities exert a favorable influence upon heart disease and that inactivity may have some deleterious effects. This is particularly true for individuals who were athletically active early in life and then suddenly limit themselves entirely to sedentary work; they run a high risk of heart attacks.

The most reasonable approach to the problem of atherosclerosis is to accept multiple factors as contributing to its development. The respective roles of the many factors, some of which were discussed above, probably vary from species to species, from race to race, and from person to person. On the basis of the foregoing discussion, the reader can probably create images of individuals most likely and least likely to suffer a heart attack from atherosclerosis of the coronary arteries. As the most likely person, picture an overweight man indulging in a fatty diet, a heavy smoker with high blood pressure and high serum cholesterol, working under emotional stress in a sedentary occupation with little outdoor activities. On the other extreme, envision a thin, wiry woman of forty, with low blood pressure and low serum cholesterol, with a family history of longevity, a placid disposition, and dietary habits involving little animal fat. It should be clear that if a group of individuals representing each type were selected and followed, there would unquestionably be some in the "most likely" group who would escape heart disease, and some in the "least likely" who would have a "coronary" heart attack, for we are dealing with probabilities and trends rather than with proven cause and effect.

The most important question of all is whether controlling any of these factors can actually be demonstrated to prevent or delay the development of atherosclerosis. Obviously, some factors are not controllable, such as heredity or hormones. Weight, tobacco, exercise, diet, and possible stress can be in part controlled. However, it is exceedingly difficult to make appropriate studies to determine conclusively the influence of changing such factors upon atherosclerosis. This is in part due to the fact that atherosclerosis is not really measurable. Two indices are widely used: (*a*) serum cholesterol (or other fatty substances in the blood), and (*b*) the frequency of heart attacks (coronary occlusion), a common, but not invariable, complication of atherosclerosis. Thus it is seen that atherosclerosis in man has to be assessed by indirect evidence which, as will be seen later, is misleading in individual cases and can be used only as mass evidence. Because of these difficulties, conclusions regarding preventibility of atherosclerosis by changes in the mode of living have to be considered with great caution. Alteration of diet presents the most controversial aspect of the prevention of atherosclerosis. As stated, dietary habits of nations or groups of individuals often parallel incidence of atherosclerosis; low serum cholesterol and low incidence of atherosclerosis are found in those whose diet is low in animal fat. Altered diets in individuals with elevated serum cholesterol, consisting of reduction of animal fats and the substitution of vegetable fats, particularly those with high content of unsaturated fatty acids, have led to a reduction of the serum cholesterol level. However, the consistency and permanence of the effective reduction of fatty compounds in the serum have not yet reached the stage where a blanket statement can be made that serum levels of cholesterol and other fatty compounds can be controlled by dietary means alone. Even if such control of blood fats were possible, one would have to assume that reduction in fat content of the blood reduces, delays, or reverses the atherosclerotic process, a conclusion which at this time appears unwarranted.

From the practical standpoint, prevention of atherosclerosis involves three major approaches: (*a*) control of diet, (*b*) elimination of some contributory factors, and (*c*) use of drugs.

Dietary recommendations have largely paralleled the evolution of the various theories derived from studies in animals and man. The earliest recommendations condemned items rich in cholesterol (eggs, butter). Later, all fats in the diet were considered undesirable. Then it was found that the fully saturated animal fats (lard, fat on meat, dairy products) may be the culprits, while unsaturated vegetable fats (corn oil, safflower oil) are not only harmless but may even be helpful in reducing serum fats. The role of sugars and starches (carbohydrates) has been questioned by some, since it became apparent that the wall of the artery can synthesize cholesterol from carbohydrates, and that carbohydrates are essential in metabolizing fats. The controversy involving the problem of diet in atherosclerosis has not been resolved, and it is generally agreed that further extensive research is needed. However, as long as there is some evidence that change in diet *may* prevent atherosclerosis and the resulting heart attacks (and strokes), thought should be given to the problem of basic rearrangement of our diets. It is clear, however, that effective reduction of serum cholesterol can be accomplished only if dietary restriction of animal fats is extreme. Such diets require very elaborate planning and preparation to be palatable and unquestionably would impose considerable hardship on the average family. Considering the unresolved questions in the matter, a committee of the American Heart Association submitted a recommendation that such diets be considered primarily in individuals who already have atherosclerosis (evidenced by a heart attack or stroke) or who have a known increase in probability of acquiring it (e.g., strong family history of heart attacks). Even then, dietary treatment of atherosclerosis has to be considered tentative and experimental rather than firmly established, and the institution of such special dietary treatment will depend on the attitude of each individual physician and patient.

The elimination of other factors is less difficult. The elimination of excess body weight and of smoking is certainly a highly desirable objective of treatment. Here, even if the relationship between these factors and atherosclerosis is equally unproved, as in the case of diet, there is strong evidence that obesity and smoking have an over-all deleterious effect upon health. The desirability of indulging in a reasonable amount of exercise is also unquestionable in terms of general health. Whether stress can or cannot be controlled is debatable, yet it is undoubtedly desirable to recommend reasonable time for relaxation to individuals engaged in highly competitive and emotionally taxing occupations. Treatment of high blood pressure will be discussed in the next chapter. Here the elimination of a contributory factor in the genesis of atherosclerosis coincides with the treatment of a disease with its own serious dangers.

Drug therapy of atherosclerosis is even more difficult to evaluate than the effect of diet. Using the serum cholesterol level as an index of drug efficacy, one has to consider the question of whether artificial reduction of serum fatty substances by drugs has any influence upon atherosclerosis. In the case of diet one at least has available observations that dietary trends in certain groups of people can be associated both with lowered serum cholesterol and lower incidence of atherosclerosis. Should future research show that the elevation of serum cholesterol and atherosclerosis are both manifestations of some over-all metabolic disease and need not be related to each other, then evidence obtained from mass observations would at least suggest the possibility that diet could control *both*. Such evidence cannot be produced for the effect of drugs lowering serum cholesterol. The number of drugs claimed to have such properties is very large: more than fifty different agents have been listed in a recent monograph on the subject. Among these are various amino acids, vitamins, unsaturated fatty acids, and many other drugs and hormones. The caution that has to be applied to the interpretation of results of tests with drugs can be illustrated by the recent experience with a powerful drug capable of lowering serum cholesterol, which had to be withdrawn from the market because of serious toxic effects upon patients. Furthermore, it was demonstrated that this drug reduced serum cholesterol at the expense of increasing other sterol compounds—a point which suggested the possibility that this type of cholesterol reduction may be irrelevant to the atherosclerotic process.

Though the various drugs have not as yet established themselves as satisfactory and proven agents, recent interest has centered around the use of hormones, namely ovarian substances and thyroid compounds, which are thought to have a possible influence on atherosclerosis. Even though the rationale here is better than that of other drugs, and the evidence by its broad general implications resembles that of dietary treatment, the practicability of long-term hormonal treatment of individuals prone to atherosclerosis has as yet not been demonstrated.

CORONARY ARTERY DISEASE

Atherosclerosis affects the entire arterial tree, but its serious consequences primarily concern the aorta and the larger arteries. Since the function of the arteries is to carry blood to distant parts of the body, this function can be interfered with only in two ways: if the wall of the arteries is so weakened that it can no longer stand the high pressure within it and ruptures; or if the disease of its wall presents obstacles to flow, interfering with or interrupting the flow of blood. Rupture of an arterial wall is rare and is mostly limited to certain portions of the aorta. The principal significant consequences of atherosclerosis thus are obstruction of the arterial lumen (lumen is space enclosed by arterial walls) and the resulting interference with the blood supply to various parts of the body. The effect of the occlusion of arteries leading to different parts of the body varies considerably. Some regions suffer more than others from occlusive arterial disease, depending upon availability of alternate channels for blood flow. Among organs most sensitive to disturbances of blood flow is the heart itself: its blood supply through the coronary arteries is generous, but such large amounts of blood are needed to provide energy for heart action that any interference with its blood supply is felt by the heart. Thus, the great need for blood supply on the one hand, and the special predilection for atherosclerotic changes to affect the coronary arteries on the other hand, make coronary disease the cardinal manifestation of atherosclerosis; its symbol, as it were.

In defining the problems of coronary artery disease it should be pointed out that atherosclerosis is not the only cause of occlusive disease of the coronary arteries. However, atherosclerosis produces such an overwhelming majority of cases of this disorder, that for practical purposes it is identified with coronary disease. Among other causes one can mention the following: (*a*) rare congenital disorders of the coronary circulation; (*b*) occlusion by emboli (clots traveling with the bloodstream from other parts of the circulation); and (*c*) obstruction of the origin of a coronary artery by syphilis (once important, now almost nonexistent). These causes are very rare and often can be suspected by virtue of the patient's age and some unusual circumstances. The ordinary manifestations of coronary artery disease thus are due to occlusive changes in these arteries produced by atherosclerosis. There is no unified terminology for these manifestations. *Coronary disease* or *coronary artery disease* is frequently used, but some prefer *coronary heart disease* or *ischemic heart disease* (ischemia— diminished blood supply). The principal manifestation of coronary disease, the "heart attack" proper, represents damage to a portion of the heart muscle. Here *coronary thrombosis* and *coronary occlusion* are used interchangeably with *myocardial infarc-*

tion, although the last term is the most correct one, signifying actual heart muscle damage.

The normal coronary circulation has been discussed in chapter 2 and shown in figure 9. It is seen that the heart is supplied with blood by three principal channels: the right coronary artery and the two major branches of the left coronary artery. Even though there are considerable individual variations as to how large a portion of the myocardium is supplied by each channel, it can be assumed that, as a rule, each artery supplies one-third of the heart muscle. The myocardium is a large user of oxygen; any deprivation of oxygen supplied by the blood may lead to damage of the delicate muscle machinery. Blood (and oxygen) deprivation, or ischemia, of the myocardium may occur in two forms: (*a*) short-term deficit, producing a temporary abnormality of the muscle wall which corrects itself when normal supply becomes available; and (*b*) long-lasting ischemia, producing permanent changes— death of the affected portion of the myocardium. The critical time separating reversible and irreversible damage to the heart muscle varies from individual to individual and is related to many factors; however, as a rule, ischemia lasting more than a few minutes causes permanent muscle changes, "wrecks the machinery," as a famous physiologist expressed it. Looking upon the problem of ischemia of the myocardium from the standpoint of occlusive atherosclerosis of the coronary arteries, one recognizes temporary, reversible myocardial ischemia in individuals in which the demand for blood supply is temporarily increased and the narrowed artery cannot keep pace with the supply. Any major obstruction in the course of the coronary artery produces long-lasting ischemia, resulting in irreversible changes in the myocardium. And yet the heart is not without defense against such a disaster.

Assuming that each major artery supplies one-third of the heart muscle, one would expect that a sudden occlusion of such an artery would bring about death to one-third of the muscle. This is not so: such an occlusion causes destruction of a much smaller portion of the muscle, usually not more than 20 percent of it. The reason for this difference is that smaller branches of the coronary arteries connect with each other and provide alternative channels of blood supply for the heart muscle. These intercoronary connections are called *collateral* channels—they are the basis for the *collateral circulation*—and are the most important defense mechanism of the heart against occlusive diseases of the coronary arteries. These collateral channels occur, under normal circumstances, only on the periphery of the coronary arteries; coronary arteries divide into branches similar to a tree, and thus it can be visualized that only peripheral branches come in close contact with branches of the next tree. The central part of the myocardium supplied by a coronary branch receives its blood exclusively from it; this is the only part damaged by its occlusion, since the peripheral portions of this area have dual blood supply. Without this collateral circulation it is unlikely that an individual would survive an attack in which 33 percent of his heart muscle were suddenly damaged beyond repair, and yet damage involving 20 percent of the myocardium can be suffered often without too many difficulties.

In addition to this protective mechanism against sudden occlusion of a coronary artery, the collateral circulation plays an even more important role when occlusion develops more slowly. These collateral interarterial branches of the coronary arteries have the capability of rapid growth and can supply more and more of the ischemic myocardium, given enough time. Thus, as an atherosclerotic plaque grows within one of the branches of the coronary artery, interfering with blood flow through it, collateral channels from the other two branches increase in size, providing effective "detours" to the ischemic area of the myocardium. Under favorable circumstances such collateral arteries can take over the entire blood supply of another artery, in which case complete occlusion of one vessel would cause no serious consequences upon the myocardium.

Coronary atherosclerosis can thus be visualized as a race between the evil, destructive forces occluding vital channels carrying blood into the heart muscle, and good, constructive forces building effective collateral channels—detours. This race can be won if the occlusive process is a slow one and if it involves primarily one coronary branch. It can be lost if it occurs too rapidly for the development of effective detours, or if the atherosclerotic process produces changes in more than one coronary branch, in which case the building of collateral channels may become difficult or even impossible.

The pathologist looks upon coronary artery disease from the standpoint of its two principal components, (*a*) atherosclerotic disease of the coronary arteries, and (*b*) consequent damage to the heart muscle. Coronary artery disease appears as plaques projecting into the lumen of the coronary arteries, as fresh thrombi (clots) usually located at points of partial occlusion of the artery by a plaque, and as scars from old thrombi. Total occlusion of a coronary artery is usually caused by a combination of thrombus and plaque. Scars from old thrombi may contract and permit the reestablishment of a narrow channel through the occluded artery (*recanalized thrombi*). Damage to the heart muscle appears in the form of fresh changes or old changes. Fresh damage is seen as softening of the heart muscle (*necrosis*); old damage as scars produced by the healing of softened areas (*fibrosis*). Both fresh and old changes may appear as large sections of damaged heart muscle (*myocardial infarction*) or as scattered areas intermingled with healthy muscle.

The clinician looks upon coronary artery disease from the standpoint of the effect of inadequate blood supply to the heart upon his patient's symptoms. It has been explained above that ischemia of the heart muscle occurs in two forms: (*a*) temporary or reversible, and (*b*) permanent or irreversible. Neither the physician nor the patient may be aware of the occlusive process in the coronary circulation if it is effectively compensated by collateral circulation. There are two major clues which draw attention to coronary disease: chest paint, which is a manifestation of ischemia of the heart muscle, and disturbance of cardiac performance, which may occur in the presence of advanced damage to the myocardium.

As a rule, chest pain reflects inadequate blood supply to the heart (see chap. 4) and lasts as long as the ischemia. Thus, temporary ischemia produces shorter attacks of pain which subside when blood supply becomes normal again; irreversible ischemia produces pain of long duration which may persist until relief is brought about by administration of drugs. Temporary ischemia is usually referred to by the clinician as *relative coronary insufficiency*. The chest pain is related to a short-term disproportion between the demand and the supply of blood to the heart. The most typical increase in demand upon the coronary circulation is produced by exercise. In the presence of relative coronary insufficiency a point is reached during the performance of exercise at which the overworked heart muscle does not receive the necessary oxygen from the blood: the patient experiences pain as a warning signal; exercise is terminated; the demands for oxygen decrease and fall within the capability of the coronary tree; ischemia is terminated and the pain ceases. This sequence of events represents the most typical manifestation of coronary artery disease, which is referred to an *angina pectoris, anginal syndrome,* or *angina of effort*. Such attacks of chest pain not only provide information that there is an obstacle within the coronary circulation, but also supply clues as to how seriously this obstacle interferes with the coronary supply to the heart. If chest pain occurs only when the exercise is unusually strenuous, then such process may be mild; if pain occurs even with minor activities, serious occlusive coronary disease may be present.

There are many modifying influences upon this typical picture of relative coronary insufficiency. Other factors than exercise may produce increased demands upon the coronary circulation. Fall in blood pressure may temporarily reduce the coronary blood supply to a point that even the resting needs of the heart cannot be met. The disproportion between coronary supply and demand may be temporarily improved by drugs such as nitroglycerin (see chap. 5). Finally, some individuals may have imperfect "warning signals" and experience little or no pain when their myocardium becomes ischemic.

In contrast to temporary myocardial ischemia, irreversible ischemia, occasionally referred to as *absolute coronary insufficiency* (in contrast to "relative") has much more profound effects upon the heart. The course of irreversible ischemia is usually complete occlusion of a coronary branch by a clot (which develops rapidly and does not allow time for collateral circulation). The irreversible damage to the myocardium appears as *myocardial infarction,* the common variety of heart attack. The average myocardial infarction involves an area of heart muscle about 3 to 5 cm. in diameter. The softened dead muscle is gradually replaced by scar tissue, a process which usually takes three to four weeks. This healing process of acute myocardial infarction coincides with the active stage of the "coronary" attack, which will be discussed later in detail. After recovery from such an attack the patient's further course depends upon two factors: (*a*) the state of the other coronary arteries; (*b*) the amount of healthy heart muscle left to perform the pumping action of the heart. Under favorable conditions recovery from acute myocardial infarction may be complete and permanent; under unfavorable circumstances myocardial infarction represents but an episode in chronic heart disease which will either lead to further attacks or to incapacity from heart failure.

It is obvious from the foregoing discussion that the physician taking care of a patient with coronary artery disease can judge its progress only from indirect evidence. Since coronary arteries are not amenable to direct examination except by the elaborate method of coronary angiography, which is not without risk and is unsuitable as a routine method for examination, the physician judges coronary disease only from its consequences upon the myocardium. He can therefore recognize the following clinical stages of coronary atherosclerosis.

STAGE I. THE ASYMPTOMATIC STAGE

Under circumstances explained above, significant coronary disease may exist without causing any signs or symptoms of disease. It is even possible to have occlusion of a major coronary artery without symptoms if collateral circulation is capable of providing 100 percent compensation for the occlusion. The widespread nature of coronary atherosclerosis in our culture makes it highly probable that the majority of men over the age of forty have some disease of the coronary arteries, though fortunately most have insignificant degrees of it.

STAGE II. RELATIVE CORONARY INSUFFICIENCY

The essence and the mechanism of relative coronary insufficiency have already been discussed. Chest pain provides a guide to the circumstances under which the disproportion between myocardial demands for oxygen and coronary blood supply develop. The principal feature of this stage of the disease is the fact that under resting conditions and during performance of activities below the level of coronary insufficiency the heart muscle is healthy. Thus, the patient may have no symptoms, there may be no abnormal findings on examination, and the electrocardiogram is usually normal under all circumstances except during periods of ischemia. During this stage the physician can often make the diagnosis by electrocardiographic changes during an exercise tolerance test (see chap. 4).

Relative coronary insufficiency varies considerably in its scope and duration. Some individuals who have normal circulatory function under most circumstances experience anginal pain only with unusually strenuous effort. At the other extreme, some patients are so close to the critical point of coronary insufficiency that they may have pain even at rest, with the slightly increased oxygen demands imposed by minor excitement. Perhaps the most crucial question in this stage of coronary disease is its over-all trend. First, the presence and degree of coronary insufficiency may be stationary: the patient has a "ceiling" to the amount of work he can perform without experiencing pain. Some individuals can live for years or decades with active coronary insufficiency and lead useful lives. Furthermore, the degree of coronary insufficiency may decrease: there may be a gradual improvement in the amount of work that can be performed without chest pain, occasionally leading to apparent cure. This is interpreted as indicative of effective building of coronary collateral "detours" by the individual. In this sense one could consider certain cases of coronary atherosclerosis "curable," which of course means only that the effective blood supply to the heart has increased, and not that coronary disease has improved. Finally, relative coronary insufficiency may become progressively worse and may be a mere transitory stage in the development of "absolute" coronary insufficiency. Unfortunately, this course is followed in many, if not most, cases of coronary atherosclerosis.

STAGE III. ABSOLUTE CORONARY INSUFFICIENCY

This irreversible form of myocardial ischemia leads to permanent destruction of a portion of the heart muscle. When this occurs, one of three things can happen: (*a*) the individual may die suddenly, usually when so much heart muscle is damaged that its function cannot be maintained; (*b*) the patient may develop the usual picture of "coronary occlusion" with myocardial infarction; (*c*) some individuals, for reasons not entirely clear, may have heart muscle destroyed without producing symptoms suggesting a heart attack, or with minor symptoms merely suggesting an "anginal attack." These patients by electrocardiogram, or at autopsy, show unmistakable evidence of having had unsuspected myocardial infarction in the past.

However, the usual sequence of events in this stage is the occurrence of coronary thrombosis with the production of the typical myocardial infarction. This manifests itself as chest pain, similar to anginal attack, but more severe, more prolonged, and not relieved by rest or by nitroglycerin. Other signs become apparent which permit the physician to recognize this as a true heart attack rather than a temporary coronary insufficiency. The features of myocardial infarction will be presented later.

STAGE IV. MYOCARDIAL DAMAGE AND HEART FAILURE

After one or more attacks of coronary occlusion with myocardial infarction some patients lose so much functioning heart muscle that the work of the heart becomes impaired. In a sense, this situation is analogous to heart failure related to chronic increase in cardiac work load, as explained in chapter 6. In the latter the heart has to perform more work because of increased demands upon the circulation. In coronary artery disease the demands upon the heart may be normal, but so much heart muscle has been destroyed by the "heart attack" that the remaining portion of the muscle must strain to perform the ordinary work load. Thus, after extensive destruction of the myocardium, patients may experience hypertrophy of the remaining portion of the heart muscle and go from a stage of compensation to decompensation—heart failure.

MYOCARDIAL INFARCTION

The mechanism of coronary occlusion with myocardial infarction has already been discussed. As one of the most important forms of heart disease, it should be presented in more detail. The immediate consequence of the total occlusion of a coronary artery is either sudden death or *severe chest pain,* previously described. In survivors, a chain of events may be initiated which make the "coronary" one of the most unpredictable of illnesses. The possible sequels and complications of acute myocardial infarction are as follows:

1) *Shock.* A certain number of individuals develop shock after coronary occlusion. Shock is due to a combination of factors: it may be related to the severe pain, it may be associated with some abnormal substances liberated from the destroyed heart muscle, it may be related to some reflexes originating in the occluded coronary arteries, or it may be a direct indication that the heart is failing and is incapable of maintaining normal blood pressure. In shock the patient exhibits low blood pressure, rapid pulse, cold perspiration, pallor, extreme weakness, and restlessness. Shock frequently develops immediately after the onset of pain, but may also be delayed by hours or even days. It is always a very serious development, although early shock which responds well to initial treatment may not affect the over-all outcome of the disease.

2) *Gastrointestinal manifestations of coronary occlusion.* Coincidentally with, or shortly after, the onset of chest pain gastrointestinal symptoms occur with great frequency. They usually consist of nausea and vomiting, which are often aggravated and perpetuated by the action of drugs administered for the control of pain (morphine, for example). The duration of nausea and vomiting is usually not long, but they may dominate the picture to such an extent that the patient has the impression that he is suffering from "indigestion" or "food poisoning" rather than a heart attack.

3) *Shortness of breath.* Shortness of breath may be a manifestation of anxiety associated with chest pain, but most often is evidence of temporary heart failure, and therefore belongs in the category of *paroxysmal dyspnea* described in chapter 4. As such it is a rather ominous occurrence, since acute heart failure would not develop unless a considerable area of muscle were destroyed. The most ominous form of dyspnea is acute pulmonary edema, which is often fatal unless immediate and vigorous action is undertaken.

4) *Arrhythmias.* Irregularities of heart action may be the most treacherous event in the course of myocardial infarction. It is known from animal experiments and observations in humans that poorly oxygenated heart muscle is more irritable and may initiate ectopic rhythms. Ventricular premature beats and ventricular tachycardia are not uncommon in the course of myocardial infarction. They may or may not affect the action of the heart, for during the critical period of cardiac weakness even slight disturbance of the normal sequence of heartbeat may be deleterious. Their significance lies, however, in their being a possible precursor of fatal ventricular fibrillation. There is no doubt that ventricular fibrillation accounts for the death of some individuals who die shortly after the onset of chest pain, perhaps before medical help can be summoned, but whose heart damage would otherwise be compatible with recovery. Ventricular fibrillation can occur any time in the course of myocardial infarction, although the most critical time for it is during the first week after

onset. Less serious forms of arrhythmias may serve as a warning and be lifesaving by alerting the medical staff to the imminence of fibrillation, so that protective measures can be instituted. Unfortunately, some patients develop ventricular fibrillation without any warning.

5) *"Constitutional reactions" to myocardial infarction.* Myocardial infarction, along with many other diseases associated with destruction of living tissue in the body, is followed by some nonspecific reactions. Among these one can include: fever, malaise, elevation of white blood cell count (*leukocytosis*), and the accelerated settling of red blood cells in the test tube (increased sedimentation rate; see under "Rheumatic Fever" in chap. 9).

6) *Heart failure.* While dyspnea may be a manifestation of acute heart failure in the immediate period after onset of myocardial infarction, it most frequently subsides, suggesting that the heart muscle was able to adapt itself to the damage. In a certain number of patients, however, persistent heart failure either follows the initial shortness of breath or develops later. The presence of heart failure in acute myocardial infarction is usually an ominous sign, although not always irreversible, suggesting extensive damage to the heart and making the probability of complete recovery somewhat less likely.

7) *Thromboembolism.* Formation of clots in the heart after myocardial infarction is a relatively common occurrence. This is due to the fact that clotting of blood inside the cardiovascular system is facilitated by the formation of rough surfaces. Myocardial infarction involving the innermost layer of the myocardium can produce roughening of the endocardium; furthermore, reduced motion of this area is an additional factor for clot formation (*mural thrombus,* or clot attached to the inner wall of the heart). These clots in no way interfere with heart action, but they can detach themselves, in part or completely, and be propelled by the bloodstream until they reach an artery which they fill snugly, occluding it and interrupting the blood flow. Such a traveling clot, or *embolus,* provides an important, often unexpected complication of myocardial infarction. The commonest emboli occur in the

brain, causing strokes, and in the legs, stopping the circulation to the leg and requiring an emergency operation. Less common emboli affect the kidneys, spleen, intestines, and the heart itself (leading to another coronary occlusion and a new infarction). Such embolic complications may develop at any time between the second and about the twentieth day after the initial attack. Their prevention is the object of anticoagulant therapy, which will be discussed later.

In addition to the threat of mural thrombi and emboli in the greater circulation, patients remaining in bed after myocardial infarction share with other immobilized patients the danger of clots forming in the veins of legs and leading to pulmonary embolism.

8) *Other consequences of myocardial destruction.* In addition to the possible unfavorable effect of myocardial infarction upon heart function, damage to the myocardium can also result in two other uncommon complications: (*a*) rupture of the heart, and (*b*) ventricular aneurysm. Rupture usually occurs when the destruction is so complete that no support can be given in a certain area (usually dead tissue is intermingled with some surviving muscle fibers). The high pressure in the ventricle can simply make the muscle totally disintegrate, and the blood can escape into the pericardial cavity. This is immediately fatal. Occasionally such rupture occurs in the ventricular septum, and an opening between the left and the right ventricle develops. Ventricular aneurysm is due to a related process: an extensive area of softened muscle may produce not rupture but a bulge, which develops on the left ventricle, resembling a blister.

The diagnosis of acute myocardial infarction can usually be made with reasonable certainty. The physician often can make a tentative diagnosis on the basis of the typical chest pain and accompanying signs and symptoms. The diagnosis is then confirmed by the electrocardiogram, which, as explained in chapter 4, is a sensitive index of damage to the myocardium. A sequence of changes in the electrocardiographic tracing, when taken at intervals of a few days, can not only establish the diagnosis but also help in indicating the location of the damage (front wall, back wall, or septal wall of the heart). The presence in the blood of specific enzymes derived from muscle destruction is also an important aid in diagnosis (see chap. 4).

Myocardial infarction is an *acute* stage of coronary artery disease, its onset signaled by the initial chest pain and its termination assumed to take place approximately four weeks afterward. This is the average period for the healing of myocardial softening (its replacement by a firm scar). Coincidentally, the frequency of the various complications decreases after the end of the second week to a point where their occurrence is considered rather remote.

THE COURSE AND TREATMENT
OF CORONARY DISEASE

Few conditions have a course as unpredictable as coronary artery disease. There are several reasons for this. In the first place, atherosclerosis in general, and coronary involvement in particular, are almost universally present in our culture. Whether or not a person has clinically significant coronary disease may merely reflect the speed of its development and the involvement of strategic arteries and thus, in a sense, represent the result of an accident. Secondly, the course of atherosclerotic involvement of the coronary tree is enhanced by complications, the most serious of which is coronary thrombosis, resulting in myocardial infarction. Thirdly, the destructive process of coronary narrowing and occlusion is counteracted by nature's repair work, whereby spontaneous healing and recovery are sometimes possible, or the progression of the process may stop at a stage tolerable for the patient.

Thus, the physician, confronted with a patient in whom he has diagnosed coronary disease, has to estimate the patient's prognosis in the light of many factors. It has been explained that coronary disease can be divided into stages. Stages II and IV involve a chronic state, Stage III an acute episode (myocardial infarction). The prognosis of myocardial infarction is unpredictable, but may provide certain guidelines which permit the division into groups with more or with less favorable outlook. As a rule, preexisting disease (e.g., hypertension, diabetes) and the evidence of severe involvement of the heart muscle by the infarction call for caution in estimating prognosis. On the other hand, previous good health and milder heart involvement permit more optimism. Statistics estimating the chances of survival of the critical four-week period in patients with acute myocardial infarction vary widely. Some series quote the immediate mortality as being as high as 30 or 40 percent; others, dealing with some selective low-risk patients, come up with figures as low as 0.5 percent. It is probably fair to say that an average patient who has a "coronary" heart attack and survives the initial hours of the attack has at least a 90 percent chance of recovery. After recovery from the attack the patient may fall into one of three categories: he may remain totally asymptomatic, reverting to Stage I of coronary disease; he may have periodic chest pain (Stage II); he may show evidence of intolerance of exercise and heart failure (Stage IV). Obviously, the first category offers the most favorable, and the third the least favorable, outlook.

Perhaps the most significant point concerning the prognosis of coronary artery disease is the fact that the very unpredictability of its course has, so to speak, two sides of the coin. While it is true that a patient in apparent good health may suddenly die or become desperately ill, it is equally true that a patient with serious manifestations of coronary disease may be totally rehabilitated for indefinite time periods. Thus coronary disease neither shares the inevitable progression and death of advanced cases of cancer, nor the continuous static disability of a wide variety of chronic systemic diseases. The example of many leading figures in politics, business, and the professions who have recovered from such serious manifestations of coronary disease as severe myocardial infarction and returned to full activity, high responsibility, and productive lives emphasizes the more optimistic side of coronary disease. And yet many injustices are being done by employers who consider the mere presence of any of the manifestations of coronary disease as a cause for automatic termination of employment or retirement. The importance of encouraging patients who have recovered from myocardial infarction, particularly those falling into better prognostic groups, to lead active and normal lives cannot be overemphasized. After all, the mental health of such individuals frequently hinges upon proper understanding of their situation; we can ill afford to subject many useful members of our society to enforced inactivity simply because they represent a higher than average statistical risk of heart attacks!

Can treatment alter the course of coronary disease? This question is one of the principal problems confronting the medical world today. Thus far, only one aspect of the problem can be provided with an affirmative answer: treatment of the acute episode in the course of coronary disease—myocardial infarction —is effective in reducing or eliminating certain complications and therefore in saving lives. The possible alteration of the over-all course of atherosclerotic disease, and coronary disease in particular, is subject to controversy, and the evidence in favor of such a favorable influence is meager and not acceptable to more cautious investigators.

The objectives of treatment of myocardial infarction are threefold: (*a*) creating favorable conditions for the best possible healing of the softened portion of the heart muscle; (*b*) encouraging the most effective compensatory phenomena: providing collateral channels to borderline areas and creating favorable circumstances for undamaged heart muscle to take over the function of the entire heart; (*c*) preventing complications.

The first two objectives involve the automatic reactions to myocardial infarction provided by nature. Relatively little can be done to influence these reactions, except to provide as complete rest as possible. Supportive treatment for impaired myocardial function is needed only in the presence of obvious heart failure. Rest for a patient during the acute episode of myocardial infarction, usually between two and four weeks, is now a standard treatment. However, concepts of rest have undergone some changes since the 1940's, for it became obvious that "complete rest" analogous to placing a broken extremity in a cast is impossible in an active organ such as the heart. Consequently, the once popular treatment of placing the patient flat in bed without any motion and spoon-feeding him is now considered more harmful than good. Less restrictive measures now used include the patient's resting comfortably in bed, able to use bedside commodes and, in some institutions, even spending a part of the day in a bedside chair.

The treatment and prevention of complications is directed against heart failure, shock, arrhythmias, and thromboembolism. Treatment of heart failure involves the usual measures described in chapter 5. Treatment of shock includes the use of oxygen, various agents for maintaining blood pressure, and other supportive measures. The presence of arrhythmias may be ominous, and even minor arrhythmias require more attention during myocardial infarction than they do in patients not acutely ill. It is presumed that less serious ventricular arrhythmias may be precursors of the dreaded ventricular fibrillation and that treatment of such arrhythmias with quinidine and procaine amide may prevent such a disaster. However, these drugs have too many undesirable effects to be used routinely in all cases. Recent advances in equipment have provided monitoring units which can instantly detect ventricular fibrillation and permit early resuscitative measures. Such measures are as yet impractical to be used routinely, but they have unquestionably saved some lives.

Treating myocardial infarction with anticoagulant drugs is a preventive measure against thromboembolism. This mode of treatment has been the subject of great controversy since its inception in 1946. Enthusiasts recommend its use in all cases of myocardial infarction; skeptics deny its effectiveness altogether. Most physicians take an intermediate view, using it in patients who they consider are more likely than the average to be subject to this complication.

The treatment of coronary disease other than during the acute episode of myocardial infarction has been discussed largely in connection with atherosclerosis, since prevention of atherosclerosis would automatically reduce or eliminate coronary disease. It has been pointed out that no effective antiatherogenic drugs have been demonstrated. The wisdom of eliminating such factors as obesity and the use of tobacco and of controlling, if possible, stress and diet has also been expounded. Control of hypertension, diabetes, and other diseases either influencing atherosclerosis or affecting the heart provides a further obvious objective of therapy. There are only two specific measures to apply to coronary disease over and above those applied to atherosclerosis as a whole: control of chest pain and the possible role of long-term anticoagulant treatment in preventing recurrences of myocardial infarction.

Control of chest pain (*angina pectoris*) involves advising patients to avoid those activities which invariably bring about pain. Drug treatment includes nitroglycerin, which is usually effective in relieving pain or in short-term prevention of an attack. Other nitrites and various other drugs are used for long-term prevention of pain, but their action is uncertain (see chap. 5). The use of long-term anticoagulant programs for patients with coronary disease is subject to even greater controversy than the use of these drugs in acute myocardial infarction. Short-term use of anticoagulant treatment in hospitalized patients is easier and safer than its use in individuals leading active lives. On the other hand, the variability and unpredictability of the course of coronary disease make the evaluation of therapeutic effectiveness difficult. The most elaborately designed mass study in England suggested that anticoagulant therapy may have a beneficial effect in young males who recovered from myocardial infarction, but only during the first year after the attack. However, even this study has been criticized by some authorities as inconclusive. The continuous use of anticoagulants in patients with clinical manifestations of coronary disease becomes a matter of the individual physician's preference.

11

Hypertension

"High blood pressure" is one of the medical terms most frequently used by laymen, and yet the connotation that it always represents a dangerous set of affairs is far from correct. In reality, the medical profession often faces a problem of separating high blood pressure as a normal human reaction to daily stresses from high blood pressure as a potentially serious disease. Even when the physician finds a persistently and severely elevated blood pressure, he may conclude that he is dealing with a "benign" type, one consistent with relatively good health for many years, rather than the fortunately rare "malignant" type of high blood pressure. The study of hypertension has seen many spectacular advances in the past two decades. Some forms of hypertension have been found to be curable by surgical operations. Many patients reap the benefit of the powerful new drugs capable of controlling high blood pressure. And yet a good deal remains to be done in this field. The cause of hypertension is still unknown in all but a handful of cases, and its prevention is not feasible. Furthermore, enough patients suffering from hypertension fail to respond to treatment or develop serious consequences in spite of treatment, that hypertension remains a major problem in the field of cardiovascular diseases.

In the normal population arterial blood pressure shows wide variation. The systolic pressure ranges from 100 to 150 mm. Hg, and the diastolic pressure from 60 to 90 mm. Hg. The upper and lower blood pressure limits quoted here are arbitrary levels, derived from measurement of a large number of healthy individuals. They cannot be considered, however, sharp cutoff points separating healthy individuals from patients suffering from "high blood pressure" or "low blood pressure." Hypertension, "high blood pressure," is considered to be significant only if persistent and repeated readings of blood pressure above the norm are found, generally much higher than the quoted minimum levels. Both abnormally high and abnormally low blood pressure are a clinical finding, a sign, not necessarily a disease. Thus, abnormally elevated blood pressure can be found under certain circumstances in healthy individuals; it can occur as a manifestation of disease elsewhere (*secondary hypertension*); it can, finally, be a persistent state, a primary disease. It is this primary disease that is the principal subject of this chapter. It is customary to refer to hypertension appearing as an independent state as *essential hypertension, hypertensive cardiovascular disease*, or *hypertensive heart disease*.

DISTURBANCES OF REGULATION OF BLOOD PRESSURE

The concept of the regulatory mechanism maintaining blood pressure at a constant level was presented in chapter 3. It was emphasized that blood pressure is maintained by a barostatic mechanism (similar to temperature regulation by thermostats), which is capable of regulating resistance at the arteriolar level by opening and closing the arterioles according to need in order to compensate for the variation in cardiac output. This pressure regulatory center is located at the base of the brain, where it receives and sends out signals via the autonomic nervous system. However, impulses sent from this center to the arterioles can be modified by chemical substances circulating in the blood, which can either strengthen or weaken the responses of the arterioles to these impulses. Thus disturbances of the pressure regulatory mechanism involving either too high or too low blood pressure can be related to one of two mechanisms: either the barostatic center is set too high or too low, so that improper nervous impulses reach the arterioles (*neurogenic mechanism*), or normal nervous impulses are improperly modified by the presence of chemical substances (*humoral mechanism*). Chemical substances that raise blood pressure by sensitizing arteriolar responses to nervous impulses are called "pressor substances"; those which desensitize responses and lower blood pressure are called "depressor agents." Such pressor and depressor effects are the properties of many chemical substances: some hormones normally produced in the body; hormones produced only under abnormal conditions; and drugs.

Disturbances of the pressure regulatory mechanism, either neurogenic or humoral, may occur temporarily or permanently. For example, temporary elevation of blood pressure may occur in normal individuals during periods of stress, anger, and excitement, presumably because of an excess of normal pressor hormones. Conversely, temporary falls in blood pressure may occur in normal individuals after prolonged standing (fatigue of regulatory center) causing faints. Furthermore, some individuals have imperfect regulation of blood pressure, which may lead to abnormal fall in blood pressure at the moment of change from lying to standing position (*postural hypotension*). Permanent disturbances of blood pressure, hypertension or hypotension, may be caused secondarily by disturbances of other organs; however, only hypertension exists as a primary, potentially serious disease. Hypotension (low blood pressure) is consistent with good health and is most frequently merely a variant of the norm, although occasionally it may be a sign of some systemic diseases (long-standing "wasting" diseases such as cancer or tuberculosis or Addison's disease).

Secondary hypertension may be related both to a neurogenic and to a humoral mechanism. The former is exemplified by certain injuries or diseases of the brain associated with high blood pressure; the latter, by elevation of blood pressure in some diseases of the secretory glands (Cushing's disease and tumors of the adrenal gland). However, the most important relationship between high blood pressure and disease of specific organs is hypertension associated with diseases of the kidneys.

HYPERTENSION AND RENAL DISEASE

The relationship between the kidney and elevation of blood pressure has been known for a long time; even before actual measurement of blood pressure was possible, astute physicians noticed that in certain diseases of the kidneys the pulse may be unusually firm and suspected high blood pressure. Not all disturbances of the kidneys produce hypertension: only in inflammatory diseases primarily affecting the filtration apparatus of the kidneys (*glomerulonephritis*) is hypertension a constant feature, both in the acute and the chronic stages. Relatively recently it has also been demonstrated that inflammation spreading to the kidney from its collecting portions (*pyelonephritis*) may also be associated with high blood pressure.

A study of the relationship between the kidney and blood pressure in experimental animals produced an interesting chapter in the search for causation of heart disease. In the early 1930's Dr. Harry Goldblatt of Cleveland found that constriction of the renal artery by a clamp produces hypertension in the dog, and removal of the clamp permits the return of blood pressure to normal. This finding created a good deal of excitement and speculation regarding causes of hypertension. Partial constriction of the artery supplying the kidney has two effects: it reduces the blood flow to the kidney (*renal ischemia*) and lowers the pressure in the artery beyond the constriction. Since the overwhelming probability was that hypertension created in this manner is of humoral origin, it was speculated that the kidney, in response to inadequate blood supply or lower pressures, or both, secretes a chemical substance which maintains the blood pressure at an abnormally high level. This was indeed an attractive theory when applied to humans, inasmuch as some kidney diseases were already known to cause hypertension. It was speculated that the kidneys might be responsible for all cases of "essential" hypertension, as one could visualize constrictive atheromatous disease, analogous to coronary artery constriction, producing effects similar to those of the "Goldblatt clamp." It was demonstrated that certain extracts of animal kidneys have properties of raising blood pressure when injected into animals and man; such substances as "renin" and the later identified "angiotensin" were isolated and shown to be powerful pressor agents. However, pathologists, examining kidneys from patients who had had severe hypertension, failed to find occluding plaques, and the theory had to be abandoned. Some skeptics even suggested that the kidney–hypertension mechanism demonstrated by Goldblatt might only be applicable to dogs (in some other animals the effect could not be duplicated) but unrelated to human hypertension. However, from time to time unusual cases were reported, such as patients who had constricted renal arteries on one side and had hypertension, and who were cured by removal of the kidney with the abnormal artery. Furthermore, rare but convincing cases of pyelonephritis involving only one kidney were found in which severe hypertension was cured by removal of the affected kidney. Thus, it became obvious that (*a*) a kidney may be the direct cause of hypertension, and its elimination may cure hypertension, and (*b*) that the Goldblatt mechanism indeed is operative in humans. In spite of these findings, the interest in renal hypertension waned, and it was generally accepted that the mechanism exists but operates rarely and has nothing to do with the common variety of *essential hypertension,* which was a disease of unknown cause.

A few years ago, however, refinements in angiography (see chap. 4) permitted detailed studies of the renal arteries during life. It became apparent that certain individuals with hypertension have constrictions of their renal arteries, which may be overlooked during post-mortem examinations. Furthermore, in a significant number of cases removal of the obstruction within the renal artery resulted in a cure of hypertension. Thus after a twenty-five year cycle the Goldblatt mechanism returned as an important cause of human hypertension. However, the recent second wave of enthusiasm may again be premature. Renal constriction, real and important as it is, still accounts for only a small fraction of cases of essential hypertension. No new proof has become available that the kidney is the culprit in other forms of hypertension. Extensive research is going on all over the world, since the cause of most cases of hypertension is still undetermined and modes of prevention are still unknown.

TYPES OF HYPERTENSION

The physician who finds high blood pressure in a patient is often confronted with a difficult problem which involves many decisions. The first two questions which he asks himself are: (1) Does this patient have hypertension? (2) If he does, what type of hypertension is it?

The first question is much more difficult to answer than one might believe. The examination of a patient by a physician involves measurement of blood pressure often under conditions of stress, inviting unusual elevation of pressure. Such blood pressure readings have been named "casual" pressure determinations, as opposed to "basal" readings, those recorded under conditions of complete rest and relaxation. The relationship of casual to basal reading varies; the former is almost always higher than the latter, but the differences between the two may be minor in some individuals, and very high in tense individuals. Thus an abnormal reading of blood pressure may simply mean an unusually high casual reading, an "overshoot" due to stress and tension in an individual who has normal pressure, perhaps, 95 percent of the time. Every physician knows that the blood pressure reading obtained when a patient is examined for the first time is usually higher, often substantially higher, than the readings obtained on subsequent examinations when the patient begins to know the physician and is more capable of relaxing. Many tense individuals, who have perfectly normal blood pressures recorded by their family physician, are found to have "high blood pressure" by other physicians, for instance examiners for insurance companies. The significance of such pressure overshoots due to tension is still a subject of controversy: some consider it an abnormal state, a precursor of future continuous hypertension; others believe it to be an innocent reaction of certain personality types. Some such "overshooters" later develop hypertension, to be sure, but this evidence is not sufficient to demonstrate that all will eventually develop hypertensive disease, and thus far no test has been designed to separate these potential hypertensives from others. It is also not known what proportion of the overshooters will become hypertensives.

Another difficulty of separating normals from abnormals lies in the blurred dividing line between the two. The slight rise of blood pressure with age makes the separation more difficult. Furthermore, some prominent authorities in the field of hypertension believe that essential hypertension is not really a disease but the end of the spectrum of normal variability. This theory takes into account the well-known familial trend to hypertension. Thus, within the general population with an over-all average systolic blood pressure reading of 125 mm. Hg there will be some families with trends of pressure levels under 100 and others with trends over 150 mm. Hg. Among the latter will be individuals whose blood pressure is higher than their inherited family trait; in such individuals a point may be reached at which high blood pressure becomes a threat to their health. The conventional view, of course, is that essential hypertension is a disease with an unknown but specific cause, which can develop in anybody but which has familial tendencies.

Assuming that the physician establishes the fact that the patient does indeed have persistent hypertension, he then has to answer the question of what type of hypertension he is dealing with. He has to place the case in one of three categories: (1) hypertension with a known cause, in which cure is possible by removing its cause; (2) hypertension with a known cause but without available cure; (3) hypertension of unknown origin (*essential hypertension*). The importance of determining to which type the patient belongs is self-evident.

1) Among "curable" forms of hypertension are the following:

(*a*) Coarctation of the aorta (to be discussed in chap. 13). Hypertension here is in part related to the mechanical obstruction of blood flow in the aorta and in part to the resulting derangement of the renal circulation (renal arteries leave the aorta below the point of obstruction). Surgical correction of coarctation cures the concomitant hypertension.

(*b*) Pheochromocytoma, tumor of the medulla (inner part) of the adrenal gland, or tumors originating from small bits of similar tissue spread along the course of the sympathetic nerves in the lower abdomen. These tumors, usually benign, manufacture large quantities of epinephrine and norepinephrine, which are normal hormones produced in smaller quantities by this tissue. Excess of epinephrine tends to cause intermittent elevations of blood pressure. The excess of norepinephrine causes persistent hypertension, indistinguishable from "essential" hypertension. Surgical removal of the tumor completely relieves the elevation of blood pressure.

(*c*) Aldosterone-producing tumors. Aldosterone is a hormone of the adrenal gland which has an important regulatory role in the excretion of salt and water. Its excess, such as exists in tumors of the adrenals composed of aldosterone-producing cells, causes significant elevation of blood pressure. Blood pressure returns to normal when the tumor is removed.

(*d*) Unilateral renal disease. It has been mentioned that pyelonephritis may be associated with hypertension. Pyelonephritis—infection of the kidney spreading from the urinary tract—almost always involves both kidneys. However, in rare cases, usually when one kidney is congenitally weak or damaged, this disease may be limited to one side. If hypertension can be proven to be related to one such diseased kidney, its removal may cure raised blood pressure. Because of the rarity of this occurrence, great caution has to be exercised in judging evidence that only one kidney is diseased before surgical treatment is recommended.

(*e*) Renal vascular hypertension. This form has already been discussed: here obstruction within the renal artery is responsible for hypertension; its relief restores normal blood pressure. It should be emphasized, however, that as a result of the present-day enthusiasm for this new field many more cases are being subjected to an operation upon renal arteries than are cured. It is true that the relationship between vascular obstruction and hypertension cannot always be demonstrated, and occasionally surgery has to be performed without convincing proof so that the patient may be given the benefit of the doubt. And yet the conservative interpretation of the results of the combined use of angiographic techniques and of chemical tests should narrow down the number of cases subjected to operations to those with a reasonably good prospect of reversal of their hypertension.

(*f*) Toxemia of pregnancy, pre-eclampsia, and eclampsia. These are stages of a relatively rare complication of pregnancy, associated with hypertension, edema, and convulsive seizures. This complication can occasionally be controlled by diet and medication, but in most severe cases associated with significant hypertension, interruption of pregnancy may become necessary. Unless the disease is permitted to go beyond the controllable stage, termination of pregnancy restores blood pressure to normal values, although some of the same women may develop permanent hypertension later in life.

(*g*) Rarely, hypertension may be associated with obstructive diseases of the urinary tract (hypertrophy of the prostate gland or kidney stones) and may be eliminated by removing the obstruction.

2) Forms of hypertension in which the probable cause is known but cannot be eliminated include the following:

(*a*) Glomerulonephritis. This type of inflammatory disease of the kidney occurs more frequently in children and is related to infections by hemolytic streptococcus in a manner similar to rheumatic fever. The acute stage of the disease is usually associated with hypertension; however, the elevation of blood pressure is related to nonrenal factors as well as to disease of the kidney. The vast majority of individuals with acute glomerulonephritis make a complete recovery, but a small proportion either enter directly into a chronic stage or develop a chronic stage later in life. These chronic forms of glomerulonephritis are almost always associated with severe hypertension, which is progressive, seldom responsive to drugs, and leads almost invariably to fatal kidney failure.

(*b*) Pyelonephritis. This form of kidney disease has already been mentioned. As stated, with very few exceptions both kidneys are affected. Pyelonephritis does not invariably cause hypertension, and the degree of blood pressure elevation varies from modest to very severe, similar to malignant hypertension. It is interesting that pyelonephritis may heal and yet permanent high blood pressure may remain.

(*c*) Cushing's syndrome. This is a complex glandular disorder involving the pituitary gland and the adrenal glands, in which overabundance of certain hormones leads to hypertension. Cushing's syndrome is in part treatable by medical or surgical means, but seldom curable.

3) Hypertension due to unknown causes is the commonest variety of elevation of blood pressure. Its recognition rests upon the finding of persistently high levels of blood pressure, particularly elevation of diastolic pressure, in which all causes listed above have been ruled out. A disease defined by the exclusion of factors rather than in a positive manner, essential hypertension may perhaps in the future be found to be due to not one but several unrelated processes. At the present time, two forms of it are generally recognized:

(*a*) Essential hypertension proper (benign hypertension), the commonest form of elevated blood pressure and an important cause of heart disease and failure.

(*b*) Malignant hypertension, which differs from benign hypertension only in degree. Here the elevation of blood pressure, particularly its diastolic level, is more pronounced. This form occurs more often in younger individuals and is less likely than benign hypertension to occur in families. It runs an accelerated course and, unless checked by early and effective treatment, leads to death within months or a very few years, usually due to kidney failure. Experts disagree on whether malignant hypertension is a separate disease or merely a more severe phase of benign hypertension. There are good arguments in favor of each view, and the issue is as yet undecided. It is a fact, however, that certain severe forms of hypertension of known origin (pyelonephritis, pheochromocytoma) may run a course indistinguishable from malignant hypertension. It would appear, therefore, that some consequences of malignant hypertension (to be described later) which provide its characteristic features may be primarily related to the very severe increase of vascular resistance due to intense spasm of arterioles.

CONSEQUENCES, DIAGNOSIS, AND COURSE OF HYPERTENSION

Prolonged elevation of blood pressure has three principal effects upon the circulatory system: (1) increased work load on the left ventricle; (2) increased "wear and tear" of the arterial system; and (3) danger that some hidden weaknesses of arterial walls will be unable to withstand the increased pressure within them.

The increase in left ventricular work is obvious, since the work is directly related to arterial pressure. Prolonged hypertension leads to left ventricular hypertrophy, which can usually compensate for the high work load for a certain length of time, but the eventual outcome is likely to be left ventricular failure (see chap. 6). Hypertension is one of the commonest, if not the commonest, cause of left ventricular hypertrophy, and the resulting heart failure is a common cause of death in hypertensive patients.

The effect of prolonged elevation of pressure upon the arterial system is twofold: "benign," less severe, prolonged hypertension tends to accelerate the atherosclerotic processes; patients with hypertension develop arterial disease earlier and in more severe form than those with normal blood pressure; women, generally resistant to the development of atherosclerotic arterial disease until after the menopause, may develop early coronary disease in the presence of persistent hypertension. Hypertension, furthermore, influences unfavorably the course of atherosclerotic coronary disease in another way: myocardial infarction is more poorly tolerated by the overloaded heart.

In malignant hypertension the spasm of the small arteries may be so intense that damage occurs to the arteries themselves and to organs supplied by them. The two organs most sensitive to damage from arteriolar spasm are the eyes and the kidneys. It is because of these secondary effects of the more severe spasm in malignant hypertension that eye and kidney changes are usually considered the distinguishing features of benign versus malignant hypertension. The eye changes consist of hemorrhages and inflammatory spots in the sensitive visual layer of the eye (retina) and of swelling of the optic disk. These ocular changes are referred to as *hypertensive retinopathy* and are usually described in terms of arbitrary grades in severity (Grades I to IV). The kidneys represent another organ sensitive to high pressure. Spasm of arterioles in the kidneys leads to permanent damage of this organ by gradually eliminating the tiny filtration units where the urine is formed. As more and more of these units are destroyed, the function of the kidney deteriorates, and eventually patients with malignant hypertension develop total kidney failure (uremia, uremic poisoning). It is noteworthy that reduction of kidney function just mentioned and the circulatory disturbances of the kidney which cause some forms of hypertension are totally unrelated to each other. Disturbances of renal circulation seldom cause failure of kidney function and, conversely, uremia (caused by factors other than hypertension) does not necessarily cause elevation of blood pressure.

The direct consequences of high blood pressure may include accidents related to rupture of blood vessels. Small hemorrhages in the conjunctivae of the eye and in the skin and other organs are of little consequence. Nosebleeds occur in hypertension and occasionally may be bothersome, difficult to control. However, the most serious consequence of vessel rupture is hemorrhages within the skull. These can occur either within the substance of the brain (*cerebral hemorrhage*) or outside the brain (*subarachnoid hemorrhage*), caused by rupture of *berry aneurysms,* small blister-like outpouchings of the wall of arteries at the base of the brain. Both types of hemorrhage are serious: cerebral hemorrhage may destroy brain substance, causing strokes; subarachnoid hemorrhage may lead to massive bleeding and death.

Another complication of hypertension, occuring most often in its malignant form and usually associated with extremely high levels of blood pressure, is the swelling (edema) of brain substance (*hypertensive encephalopathy*), which may lead to violent headaches, disturbances of brain function, and coma. Hypertensive encephalopathy constitutes, as a rule, an acute crisis, which may be fatal but which is usually amenable to treatment.

The *diagnosis* of hypertension may present some difficulties. First, the fact must be established that significant and persistent hypertension is present, rather than that elevation of blood pressure is transient. Then, it is necessary to attempt to find its cause. Finally, the stage of the disease and its consequences have to be assessed.

The difficulty of separating casual elevations of blood pressure from true hypertension has already been discussed. It is always necessary to make repeated measurements of blood pressure, preferably under a variety of circumstances. Some physicians prefer to hospitalize patients and take frequent measurements of their blood pressure over a 24-hour period; others observe the patients under a variety of conditions; still others study the effect of various agents which may lower or elevate blood pressure (use of sedatives, immersion of the patient's hand in ice water). The most convincing evidence that hypertension is a real problem in a given patient is the detection of one of the consequences of hypertension, such as enlargement of the heart, evidence of left ventricular hypertrophy in the electro-cardiogram, or changes in the eye grounds.

When there is reasonable evidence that the elevation of blood pressure is significant and is a disease state, then the physician has to consider the possibility that the hypertension may be due to one of the curable causes. The probability of finding curable hypertension is low, less than 5 percent. Yet the possibility—even remote—of finding a complete cure for a patient with a serious disease of the circulatory system justifies a most careful survey. The search for curable forms of hypertension involves a meticulous physical examination, the use of X rays and various laboratory procedures, and some highly specialized techniques. These include test doses of various drugs; elaborate chemical tests of the blood and urine; function tests of the two kidneys separately, which require special urological techniques; the use of radioisotopes; and the contrast visualization of the renal arter-ies. The expense of such tests is considerable, and there is some risk involved in their application; their routine use in every patient found to have elevated blood pressure is both impractical and ill advised. The physician has to discriminate by selecting patients in whom the probability of finding a curable mechanism is higher than average. The selection of patients for an extensive "work-up" requires experience and good judgment on the part of the physician.

The assessment of the stage of the disease and its conse-quences for the circulatory system and other organs is the third step in the diagnosis. Such a survey is of considerable impor-tance in the ordinary forms of "essential" hypertension, as it con-stitutes the basis for the selection of proper treatment for the patient. This will be discussed later.

The *course* of hypertensive disease is quite variable. Disability and death usually occur as a result of the following causes: (*a*) heart failure, (*b*) coronary disease, (*c*) cerebral hemorrhage or thrombosis, and (*d*) renal failure. The implications are that the fate of a patient with hypertension depends upon three factors: (*a*) how severe and persistent is the elevation of blood pressure, (*b*) how well can the heart and the vascular system resist the increased work and the wear and tear, (*c*) how successful is treatment. The assessment of these factors by the physician is only very crude and incomplete. The most important reason for this is the lack of knowledge of how persistent and severe the blood pressure elevation is over the 24-hour period in a given patient. In the future, it is hoped, it may become possible to study consistently the continuous level of blood pressure by means of automatic recording devices, which are now being tested but are not as yet widely available and applicable. The effect of treatment is variable, resulting in many brilliant successes but also in some failures. Within the course of hypertension there seems to be a "point of no return," after which treatment is no longer effective. This is particularly true in cases in which renal function is already impaired.

Many patients with hypertension, even of severe degree, lead active lives and often are completely unaware of their condition. This is due to the fact that elevation of blood pressure in itself need not in any way interfere with the person's health. Symptoms are usually related to the consequences of high blood pressure rather than to elevation of blood pressure per se. Two widely known symptoms, headaches and the sensation of pounding of the heart, occur in hypertension less commonly than is generally believed and are often unrelated to its severity. Physicians caring for patients with high blood pressure are aware of many seeming paradoxes. On the one hand, certain individuals, particularly women after menopause, can carry blood pressures as high as 250/120 for many years without apparent ill effects, even when no treatment is given. On the other hand, some patients with much more modest elevation of blood pressure develop heart failure and die. The play of the aforementioned factors probably accounts for these differences.

The course in benign hypertension is entirely different from that in its malignant form. The former, which accounts for the great majority of cases, often persists for many years, permits an active and asymptomatic life for long periods of time, and may be permanently controllable by medication, similar to the control of diabetes. Malignant hypertension, on the other hand, has a rapidly progressive course and may lead to disability or death within a short time. Until modern methods of treatment were introduced, malignant hypertension was invariably fatal. Even now, only a certain portion of cases is controllable, others having reached the irreversible stage before effective treatment could be instituted.

TREATMENT OF HYPERTENSION

The introduction of new drugs in the treatment of hypertension has provided one of the dramatic advances in medicine and has profoundly affected the course of the disease. Hypotensive therapy, however, is not new. For many years, various drugs were claimed to have blood pressure-reducing properties. Most of those are now considered ineffective, and their earlier successes were unquestionably due to the difficulty of separating drug effects from fall in blood pressure occurring from other causes. Since blood pressure is a body function influenced by many factors, including daily stresses, reduction of blood pressure can be accomplished by many nonspecific means, such as the decrease in body weight, the reduction of number of working hours, and the introduction of relaxing diversification, or vacation. Mild sedatives have been used successfully for many decades in the treatment of hypertension, although such drugs have no relationship whatsoever to blood pressure-regulating functions and merely help the individual to relax and relieve his tension. These general measures are still widely used and constitute an important part of modern therapy, particularly in milder cases and in patients suspected of being merely "overshooters."

Specific means for control of blood pressure can, on theoretical ground, be directed against the nervous and humoral factors involved in high blood pressure (see above). Since the nervous control of blood vessels is indicated by the autonomic nervous system, and since its sympathetic part has blood vessel-constricting properties, an operation was designed, in the 1930's, to interrupt sympathetic nerves supplying the thoracic and the abdominal organs and the lower extremities, in the hope of relaxing permanently the constricted arterioles in hypertensive patients. This operation, *sympathectomy,* has undergone many modifications, involving resections of larger or smaller parts of the sympathetic nerves, and has produced considerable controversy regarding its efficacy. There appear to have been a number of cases with genuine reversal of severe hypertension, particularly following the more radical forms of sympathectomy. And yet most cases, according to more cautious investigators, showed inconclusive results, which could perhaps have been produced by the nonspecific means discussed above.

A search for effective drugs proceeded along three principal lines: (*a*) the possibility of finding a specific chemical substance which would neutralize and counteract the humoral agent (angiotensin?) involved in the causation of certain forms of hypertension; (*b*) a search for an effective chemical which would block sympathetic nerve impulses, thus performing a "nonsurgical sympathectomy"; (*c*) the exploration of changes in body electrolytes, which may have effects upon pressure control. No conclusive strides occurred along the first line of investigation; some claims have been made concerning certain drugs, but these have not been substantiated, nor were results of such treatment impressive. However, the search for drugs affecting the autonomic nervous system resulted in the major breakthrough in the treatment of hypertension. The first drug from this series was hexamethonium, a relatively simple chemical compound, which is only effective by injection and has a short period of action, so that repeated injections had to be given during the day. Awkward and impractical as this drug was, it nevertheless provided the first conclusive proof that drug therapy could control blood pressure in certain severe forms of hypertension. Afterwards, a variety of similar drugs were developed which were effective in tablet form and had longer active properties. Most of these belong to the category of *ganglionic blockers,* drugs interrupting the transition of impulses at the ganglions (a group of cells at the junction of nerves). Since the autonomic nervous system has many other functions besides regulating the size of arterioles, such blocking agents produce many other manifestations in addition to reduction of blood pressure, most of which are undesirable (constipation, blurred vision, difficulty in urination). These "side effects" of such hypotensive drugs often limit their use. A search for an "ideal" hypotensive drug which would specifically reduce blood pressure without influencing other functions has not yet been fulfilled, but such an agent is theoretically possible.

Many other effective drugs are now available which are better tolerated than ganglionic blockers and, though less effective, provide an important part of treatment of benign hypertension. Among those are drugs derived from plants (rauwolfia serpentina, veratrum viride); the chemical agent, hydralazine, which was originally thought to be an antihumoral–pressor agent; some tranquilizers from the series of mono-amino oxidase inhibitors; and, most recently, another enzyme inhibitor, alphamethyl DOPA. Among the most important hypotensive drugs are derivatives of the diuretic chlorthiazide, which control water and electrolytes. These drugs are most effective when used in conjuction with other hypotensive agents. Their importance lies in making some weaker hypotensive drugs more potent and permitting the reduction of the effective dose of ganglionic blockers and other powerful agents, thereby making them more tolerable for the patient. The mode of reduction of blood pressure of the chlorthiazide series is not entirely understood; their effect upon the elimination of salt and water in the body may reduce the blood volume (and cardiac output). The action of chlorthiazide diuretics is probably analogous to the effect of a low-salt diet, which was once very popular in the treatment of hypertension. Such diets, although helpful and even dramatic in a certain number of patients, required such extreme limitation of the variety of food (for example, rice and fruits only) in order to be effective that it was incompatible with leading an otherwise normal life and therefore was limited in application. The introduction of modern hypotensive drugs has made the use of such extreme dietary restriction obsolete.

Because of the great variety of agents available for the therapy of hypertension, such treatment requires a great deal of skill and thought on the part of the physician. He has many courses of action to choose from:

1) He may elect no treatment at all, assuming that a certain high blood pressure reading does not represent the *disease,* hypertension, but merely excitement on the part of the patient.

2) He may limit himself to the use of nonspecific methods of treatment: reduction of body weight, regulation of the patient's working conditions with shorter hours and longer periods of rest and relaxation, and, perhaps, the addition of mild sedation.

3) He may institute active hypotensive therapy with milder drugs, aiming at a dosage and combination of drugs best suited to this case, but limiting himself to agents which in no way interfere with the patient's life and require relatively little control.

4) He may find it necessary to use the powerful hypotensive drugs, which usually require strict supervision and frequently make the patient miserable.

The foregoing discussion deals exclusively with therapy of the blood pressure elevation. In the course of hypertension, there are many other problems which require treatment, particularly the various sequels and complications of hypertension. They add to the complexity of the problem of control of high blood pressure, which represents one of the major challenges to medicine.

12

Diseases Affecting the Valves of the Heart

Malfunction of valves of the heart produces disturbances of the heart and circulation which range from insignificant abnormal "noises" in the heart to serious, even fatal afflictions. Since surgical treatment of mitral stenosis became available in 1948, this field has been entirely dominated by cardiac surgery. At first, obstructive diseases of the valves could be relieved by relatively simple operations; then open-heart surgery offered opportunities to correct other forms of valve malfunctions; finally replacement of a defective valve with an artificial prosthesis produced the "ultimate" in surgical treatment of valve disease. And yet, a sober look at the results of such operations reveals that they are far from being the final answer to the problem. The risk is still appreciable; the long-term fate of artificial valves has yet to be determined; the functioning of artificial valves offers a great improvement over the functioning of diseased valves, but does not as yet approximate normal valve function. Consequently, the presence of valve disease does not automatically imply surgical treatment. Thorough evaluation of each patient has to be made and cases most suitable for operative treatment carefully selected. Each deformity of a valve produces a specific pattern, which is explained in this chapter. The thorough knowledge of such patterns facilitates the prediction of a patient's fate, and hence permits the separation of patients who can best be treated medically from those who need operations.

TYPES AND CAUSES OF VALVE DISEASE

Each of the four cardiac valves can be altered in two ways: it can become incapable of opening completely so that the orifice is narrowed (*stenosis* of the valve); or its function as a valve may be impaired by incomplete closure, producing *insufficiency* of the valve, through which the blood regurgitates in the wrong direction. Diseases of the cardiac valves are commonly acquired during life, though some represent congenital malformations. Three valves—the mitral, aortic, and tricuspid valves—are more often subject to acquired diseases; stenosis of the fourth—the pulmonary valve—is almost always congenital.

There are several causes of valve deformities, but the commonest by far is *rheumatic fever*. Residual damage from rheumatic fever accounts for most cases of mitral stenosis, a majority of cases of mitral insufficiency, and for a significant number of cases of aortic stenosis and insufficiency.

Both stenosis and insufficiency of a cardiac valve vary considerably in degree. The effect of valve deformity and its malfunction is increased work load upon the heart. Such increased load may be insignificant, moderate, or severe, with circulatory consequences varying accordingly. As a general rule, reduction of a valve orifice to one-half its original size produces no significant consequences whatsoever. When the obstruction exceeds one-half of the orifice a murmur becomes apparent, but significant increase in work load does not develop until the obstructed valve approaches one-quarter of the original size. Similarly, it requires an appreciable amount of regurgitation through an incompetent valve in order to produce significant cardiac overwork, even though characteristic murmurs appear with a much less than significant degree of regurgitation. The field of valvular heart disease has undergone drastic change in recent years because (*a*) quantitative determination of the functional status of valves has become possible, and (*b*) surgical correction or replacement of faulty valves has permitted observations on the regression of changes caused by valve disease.

MITRAL STENOSIS

Mitral stenosis is almost always caused by rheumatic fever. Acute rheumatic fever (see chap. 9) frequently produces changes in the mitral valve which at first may have no effect upon its function, or which may cause mild mitral valve insufficiency. After a patient's recovery from the acute attack there may be a period of years during which no detectable effect or only minor effect upon the mitral valve is apparent. The process, which eventually leads to obstructive disease of the mitral valve, consists of a scar formation whereby the valve tissue shrinks and grows together. Consequently, five or ten years after the attack mitral stenosis may become apparent.

As explained in chapter 2, the mitral valve consists of two leaflets which open and close, aided by the chordae tendineae. The scarring process after healing of acute rheumatic fever has a tendency to join the two mitral valve leaflets, forming two mitral *commissures,* as shown diagrammatically in figure 25c. Thus, the commonest type of mitral stenosis is the fusion of the two leaflets, reducing the size of the open valve, so that, instead of a wide orifice, only a relatively small hole in its center remains open for movement of blood. The deformed, scarred valve is a favorite spot for the deposition of calcium: calcified mitral valves become even stiffer, the obstruction to blood flow becomes more pronounced. Mitral stenosis, thus, not only represents a late effect of rheumatic fever developing after years of complete absence of any detectable valve deformity, but once present it may become gradually progressive, leading to more and more obstruction with increasingly serious effects upon the circulation. The consequences of mitral stenosis upon the circulatory system are as follows:

1) Milder degrees of valvular obstruction may produce the characteristic murmur of mitral stenosis but have no disturbing effect upon the circulation of blood.

2) When the mitral valvular obstruction reaches a certain

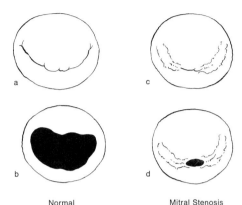

Normal   Mitral Stenosis

FIGURE 25. *Diagrammatic presentation of the mitral valve viewed from left atrium.*

a. Normal mitral valve is shown by two leaflets, one large and one small, which close the orifice completely.

b. Normal mitral valve, open widely during diastole.

c. In mitral stenosis peripheral parts of the mitral valve are joined together at the commissures. However, in systole the valve can close completely.

d. In mitral stenosis only a small central part of the mitral valve is capable of opening during diastole, producing severe obstruction of the orifice.

critical degree (usually about one-third the original size of the mitral orifice), then the flow of blood through the mitral orifice requires more expenditure of energy, as shown by a difference in pressure on the two sides of the valve: the pressure in the left atrium, which is ordinarily identical with the pressure in the left ventricle during the ventricular filling period, becomes *higher* than that in the ventricle. This difference in pressure, called a *pressure gradient,* gives a rough index of the severity of stenosis: the higher the gradient, the more severe valve stenosis. Thus, when normally both pressures (left atrium and left ventricle in diastole) are about 5 mm. Hg, in mild mitral stenosis left atrial pressure measures 10 to 15 mm. Hg, in moderate stenosis 20 to 25 mm. Hg, and in severe stenosis 30 mm. Hg and more, while the diastolic pressure in the left ventricle remains normal at 5 mm. Hg. Pressure gradients are accentuated by factors causing increased flow of blood (such as excitement and exercise) and minimized by diminished blood flow (heart failure, causing low cardiac output). Thus it is seen that the immediate effect of mitral stenosis is the elevation of pressure in the left atrium.

3) This elevation of pressure in the left atrium causes its enlargement and hypertrophy. While atrial hypertrophy does not have the same significance as hypertrophy of ventricles with its production of heart failure, such changes in the left atrium may lead to important complications, which will be discussed later.

4) The consequences of high pressure in the left atrium are identical with those caused by left ventricular failure (see chap. 6): pressure in the pulmonary veins rises, in turn causing higher pressure in the pulmonary artery and the right ventricle. The obstruction to flow at the mitral orifice acts as a dam: blood dams up under higher pressure in the lungs and causes an increased quantity of blood to remain in the pulmonary circulation. The lungs, filled with more blood, under higher pressure, become stiffer and require more effort to move during respiration, and the patient then becomes aware of an increased effort in breathing; he experiences shortness of breath.

5) Increased pressure in the pulmonary artery means an increased work load upon the right ventricle. This is occasionally aggravated by constriction of the pulmonary arterioles, producing further increase in pulmonary artery pressure—pulmonary hypertension. The increased work load upon the right ventricle eventually leads to its failure, producing edema and other manifestations already described.

Thus, the direct effects of mitral stenosis are: increased pressure in the left atrium; its increased size; pulmonary hypertension and pulmonary congestion; right ventricular hypertrophy and right ventricular failure. The patient's significant symptoms include shortness of breath and, later, edema.

Closely associated with these consequences of mitral stenosis are its important complications:

1) *Atrial fibrillation.* The increased size of the left atrium and increased pressure within it are the most powerful and consistent factors producing atrial fibrillation. Atrial fibrillation is extremely common in mitral stenosis: it occurs in more than half of all cases, and in about three-quarters of cases of severe mitral stenosis. The large left atrium perpetuates this form of arrhythmia, so that its treatment is often unsuccessful. Atrial fibrillation has two important influences upon the course of mitral stenosis: it limits the efficiency of cardiac performance, thereby aggravating the disability caused by mitral stenosis; and it facilitates the formation of clots upon the wall of the atrium, which constitute dangerous sources of emboli.

2) *Emboli in the systemic circulation.* Mitral stenosis complicated by atrial fibrillation is, as stated above, a common source of emboli (clots traveling with the circulation and settling in distant organs). The most dangerous emboli are those affecting the brain, which may cause temporary or permanent strokes, and those affecting the extremities, which may necessitate emergency operations.

3) *Pulmonary edema.* This ominous form of dyspnea, described in connection with heart failure, occurs occasionally in mitral stenosis and may be fatal. The high pressure in left atrium and in the lungs constitutes the background for this complication.

4) *Pulmonary hemorrhage.* High pressure in the pulmonary circulation, particularly in the pulmonary veins, may cause occasional rupture of a small vessel in the lungs and produce pulmonary hemorrhage. This may range from bringing up blood-tinged sputum to expectoration of large quantities of blood (as much as a cupful). However, such hemorrhages are seldom so serious as to produce anemia or necessitate blood transfusion.

The course of mitral stenosis is variable. In milder cases, the life-span of a patient may be entirely undisturbed, and mitral stenosis may merely manifest itself by the presence of murmurs and minor, nondisabling symptoms. Severe cases may cause serious disability early in life and necessitate surgical intervention in the twenties, or even earlier. A typical case of mitral stenosis can be summarized as follows: a woman (women outnumber men about three to one in the incidence of mitral stenosis) had one or more attacks of rheumatic fever in childhood, but had no difficulty after recovery and led a normal life, even though she knew that she had a heart murmur. She went through three pregnancies with only minor difficulties. In her late thirties she suddenly went into heart failure coincidentally with the development of a rapid, irregular heartbeat (atrial fibrillation). Heart failure was overcome by medical treatment, but the patient never regained the ability to perform all desired activities and found herself moderately disabled. Then the mitral stenosis was surgically treated, and the patient was considerably improved.

This illustrative case emphasizes that disability more often develops abruptly than gradually. This may be the result of atrial fibrillation or, less frequently, other factors which place extra burden upon the circulation: severe intercurrent infection, overexertion, pregnancy, and so on. Disability which develops after such an incident may be stationary or may become progressively worse. A patient's condition may deteriorate as a result of increasing pulmonary hypertension, which eventually leads to right ventricular failure.

The course of mitral stenosis has been materially altered by the introduction of surgical relief, used consistently since 1948 (earlier successful attempts were made, but only sporadically). However, surgical treatment of mitral stenosis, to be discussed later, does not mean reestablishment of a normal mitral valve, even when an artificial valve is used to replace the diseased valve, and one can only think in terms of improvement, sometimes only temporary, rather than "cure" of mitral stenosis.

The *diagnosis* of mitral stenosis is made on the basis of the characteristic murmur, changed heart sounds, enlargement of the left atrium as seen in the X ray and electrocardiogram, and other clinical signs. The severity of mitral stenosis can be assessed by the degree of the patient's disability. However, such assessment may be deceptive, because occasionally patients suffer appreciably in spite of a relatively mild degree of obstruction of the mitral valve, while others can tolerate quite severe narrowing of the valve without much interference with their lives. The clinician can often estimate the degree of stenosis on the basis of certain clinical findings, but the "ultimate" in assessing mitral stenosis is cardiac catheterization, in which it is usually possible to estimate the actual available size of the mitral orifice and to measure its effect upon the circulation as a whole, and the pulmonary circulation in particular.

Treatment of mitral stenosis can be divided into two stages: medical and surgical. Medical treatment cannot directly influence the development or progression of the obstruction of the valve, but its objective is threefold: (*a*) to prevent a recurrence of rheumatic fever, which could further damage the valve (see chap. 9); (*b*) to control activities, regulate the mode of living, and eliminate factors which could unfavorably influence the circulatory apparatus; (*c*) to prevent and treat complications. Within the scope of the last category are included: the restoration, if possible, of sinus rhythm in patients who developed atrial fibrillation, or the control of ventricular rate in untreatable atrial fibrillation; the use of anticoagulants in patients who had emboli, in order to prevent recurrences.

Surgical treatment involves three methods; the simplest and oldest attack upon mitral stenosis is the "closed" mitral valvulotomy. This operation consists of inserting the finger through a small hole in the atrium into the beating heart and fracturing the commissures binding together the two mitral leaflets. This action can be reinforced by an instrument used to "crack" tough valves. The second method is the "open" mitral valvuloplasty, in which the patient is connected with a heart-lung machine, the circulation through the heart stopped, and the valve repaired under direct vision. The third method, which also involves open-

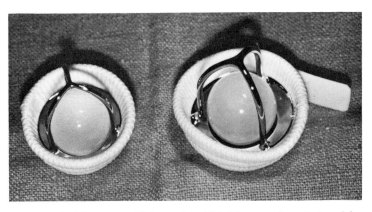

FIGURE 26. *The most widely used artificial heart valve, designed by Starr and Edwards, shown here in two sizes. The valve consists of a collar which is sewn into the heart, a steel cage, and a plastic ball. Average diameter of the ball is 2 cm.*

heart surgery, consists of replacing the valve with an artificial valve, the most widely used of which is a ball valve in a metal cage, designed by Starr and Edwards (fig. 26). There is a considerable difference of opinion about the respective merits of the three methods, but as a general rule the first carries the smallest, and the third the highest, risk. In carefully selected cases there is a proper place for each of these operations. The decision for or against surgical treatment varies considerably in different cardiac centers of our country. As a general rule, patients are selected because of appreciable disability and unresponsiveness to medical treatment, particularly when their symptoms are becoming progressively worse.

MITRAL INSUFFICIENCY

Deformities of the mitral valve producing insufficiency of the valve through which the blood regurgitates into the left atrium are due to a number of causes, in contrast to mitral stenosis, which is almost always due to rheumatic fever. Rheumatic heart disease accounts for some cases of mitral deformity; others may have been present since birth (congenital) or may represent residual changes from an attack of bacterial endocarditis or may be due to rupture of the anchoring valve cords (chordae tendineae) from known or unknown causes. In addition, mitral insufficiency may be caused by undue stretching of the orifice without any deformity of the valve. This occurs, secondarily to heart failure, with marked dilatation of the left ventricle. Rheumatic mitral insufficiency differs from rheumatic mitral stenosis in that the valve becomes incompetent during, or immediately after, an acute attack of rheumatic fever, while in stenosis the scarring process produces obstruction years afterwards.

Mitral insufficiency has a wide range of consequences upon the circulatory system. Mild mitral insufficiency may be totally insignificant and may have no untoward effects whatsoever upon the circulation. Moderate mitral insufficiency produces a variable degree of disability in a manner similar to mitral stenosis. Severe mitral insufficiency may be extremely serious, and may rapidly lead to heart failure. In this respect mitral insufficiency is potentially more serious than mitral stenosis, since the latter is produced by a chronic, gradual process and the former may appear suddenly.

The circulatory consequences of mitral insufficiency are as follows: the left ventricle, while pumping blood into the aorta, "loses" blood, which regurgitates back into the atrium with each contraction; this causes a considerable increase in the left ventricular work load. For example, if each ventricular contraction ejects the normal amount of 75 cc. of blood into the aorta, and if an equal amount leaks back, the work load of the left ventricle doubles. Cases in which an equal amount flows forwards and backwards constitute only moderate mitral insufficiency, for it has been shown that in some patients three times as much blood is regurgitated into the atrium as is ejected into the aorta! Increased work load for the left ventricle leads to its hypertrophy and may eventually produce its failure. In addition, high pressure in the left ventricle is transmitted through the incompetent valve back into the left atrium. Increased pressure in the left atrium produces consequences similar to those of mitral stenosis: dilatation, hypertrophy of the left atrium, and increased pressure in the pulmonary circulation, leading to right ventricular overload and then failure. Mitral insufficiency may also produce atrial fibrillation with its possible consequences: thrombi in the atrium and emboli in the systemic circulation.

The course of mitral insufficiency is somewhat similar to that of mitral stenosis except for the more serious nature of severe mitral insufficiency. As already indicated, it may appear early in childhood during or immediately after acute rheumatic fever. Like mitral stenosis, moderate mitral insufficiency can be well tolerated for many years. Onset of disability is often brought about by the development of atrial fibrillation.

The *diagnosis* of mitral insufficiency can be made easily by the physician on the basis of heart murmur and other findings evident on physical examination. The estimation of its severity is easier than in mitral stenosis. Mitral insufficiency increases the work load of the left ventricle; hence, the size and performance of the left ventricle provide a reasonable index of the severity of the disease. On the other hand, cardiac catheterization is less reliable in the diagnosis of mitral insufficiency. Regurgitation through the mitral valve can be only indirectly deduced from the findings of cardiac catheterization, in contrast to mitral stenosis, in which the degree of obstruction can be accurately measured. Special methods of study have been devised, such as dye dilution methods and angiocardiography with injection of the contrast substance into the left ventricle. However, even these methods provide only rough indices, rather than true measurements of mitral insufficiency. Yet cardiac catheterization does play an important role in evaluation of mitral insufficiency, for it permits the assessment of its consequences upon the circulation, particularly its effect upon the left ventricle, upon the pulmonary circulation, and upon the right side of the heart.

Treatment of mitral insufficiency consists of medical and surgical means and resembles that of mitral stenosis. In cases with clear-cut evidence for rheumatic origin of mitral insufficiency, preventive treatment for rheumatic recurrences is indicated. Other steps include warnings against overexertion, reduction of potential factors imposing strain on circulatory apparatus (overweight, anemia), and treatment or control of atrial fibrillation and its complications.

Surgical treatment of mitral insufficiency differs considerably from that of mitral stenosis. There is no simple "closed-heart" operation, so that all cases require open-heart surgery. Several methods are used for the repair of incompetent mitral valves under direct vision, but they are effective only in certain types of valvular deformities. Many, perhaps most, cases require replacement of the damaged valve with an artificial prosthetic valve. High probability that the natural valve will have to be replaced makes the over-all risk of surgical treatment considerably greater than in mitral stenosis; consequently, more conservatism has to be used in the selection of cases for surgical treatment. In most cardiac centers only patients with a considerable degree of progressive disability are considered suitable candidates for surgical treatment.

AORTIC STENOSIS

The development of aortic stenosis is in some respects similar to that of mitral stenosis, but also shows important differences. Like mitral stenosis, aortic stenosis is a slowly progressive lesion which may be the result of fusion (growing together) of valve leaflets. However, unlike mitral stenosis, the most important mechanism producing obstruction to blood flow is not the fusion but the stiffening of the valve leaflets by calcium deposit. The common type of aortic stenosis is thus *calcific aortic stenosis*. Calcium deposits do not form upon valves unless they have previously been damaged and deformed. The two most important causes of such background damage are: (*a*) congenital bicuspid valve (aortic valve formed before birth with two rather than three leaflets), and (*b*) deformity and fusion due to rheumatic

fever. Calcium deposition upon the valves takes place very slowly, so that the aortic orifice is very gradually obstructed. In
mitral stenosis scarring and valve obstruction often reach a
stable, nonprogressive stage, but in aortic stenosis the lesion
usually becomes worse with time.

Aortic stenosis affects the dynamics of heart action by producing a resistance to the ejection of blood from the left ventricle
into the aorta. Mild obstruction may merely cause a murmur;
significant obstruction raises pressure within the left ventricle in
order to overcome the resistance to ejection of blood. This
occurs when the orifice is reduced to about one-quarter of the
original opening. Thus, systolic pressure in the left ventricle and
in the aorta are no longer the same: left ventricular systolic
pressure rises above that in the aorta; the difference in pressure
between them (pressure gradient) is an index of the severity of
obstruction. In severe aortic stenosis the gradient may reach 150
or 200 mm. Hg, so that in order to maintain a normal arterial
pressure of 100 mm. Hg, the pressure in the left ventricle has to
rise in systole to 250 mm. Hg or higher. As a result of such
elevation of pressure in the left ventricle its work load is greatly
increased, an effect similar to severe hypertension. However,
there is one important difference between aortic stenosis and
hypertension. In the latter the increased demands upon the coronary circulation caused by the high work load of the ventricle
are met by a corresponding increase in pressure in the aorta,
which forces more blood into the coronary arteries. In aortic
stenosis demands for increased coronary flow are just as great
as in hypertension, because of comparable pressure in the ventricle; however, the *lower* (normal) pressure in the aorta cannot
drive sufficient blood into the coronary circulation to meet these
demands, and consequently the heart is undersupplied with
blood. This has an important bearing upon the course of aortic
stenosis.

The course of aortic stenosis is different from that of mitral
valve disease. In the first place, left ventricular overload can be
compensated by hypertrophy of the left ventricular muscle for

a good many years. Disability due to shortness of breath is uncommon, and appears quite late in the course of aortic stenosis. In the second place, the average age of development of significant obstruction of the aortic valve is higher than in mitral disease. Even though serious symptoms of aortic stenosis, both congenital and that caused by rheumatic diseases, may occasionally occur in the twenties or thirties, the characteristic age of "trouble" from aortic stenosis is the fifties and sixties. Here men outnumber women, though not by as high a ration as the reverse is true in mitral stenosis. In the third place, aortic stenosis produces certain dangerous and ominous symptoms which are unique for it and are not related directly to increased left ventricular work load and failure. These are: (*a*) chest pain, resembling anginal pain, from coronary insufficiency; (*b*) attacks of dizziness; and (*c*) sudden loss of consciousness. These symptoms are related to the aforementioned difficulties in obtaining adequate coronary circulation and, perhaps, to inadequate circulation through the brain. Both chest pain and loss of consciousness may result in death, and a certain number of patients with aortic stenosis die suddenly under such circumstances, sometimes with very little warning. In spite of the fact that the actual number of such fatalities is small, the possibility of sudden death in a person seemingly well has to be considered in anyone suffering from moderately severe or severe aortic stenosis when risks of surgical treatment are weighed.

The *diagnosis* of aortic stenosis is based, along with other valve defects, primarily on the characteristic findings detected on physical examination. Its severity can be roughly estimated by the degree of left ventricular hypertrophy, by certain characteristics of the pulse, and by other indirect means. However, the exact determination of its severity is based on physiological measurements obtained during cardiac catheterization of the left side of the heart. In the over-all evaluation of a patient with aortic stenosis difficulties may arise in the interpretation of chest pain. Patients are in the age group in which coronary disease is common, and consequently it may not be possible to determine whether the pain is caused by aortic valve obstruction or by coincidental coronary atherosclerosis. This point is a crucial one when surgical treatment is being considered, since aortic valve surgery can relieve the obstruction, but will not necessarily be beneficial in coronary disease. It is sometimes necessary to make an angiographic examination of the coronary arterial tree in order to settle this point.

Treatment of aortic stenosis has relatively little to offer short of surgical relief. There is no way in which chest pain, dizziness, or loss of consciousness can be influenced by medical treatment, except by advising patients to avoid undue physical effort. Shortness of breath and other symptoms of heart failure are considered urgent indications for surgical treatment. In cases where such treatment is for some reason not done, patients are customarily treated for heart failure.

Surgical treatment of aortic stenosis consists almost entirely of open-heart surgery. Closed relief by means of instruments advanced blindly into the aortic orifice in an effort to separate the fused valve leaflets has been done in the past, but has largely been abandoned because of the very low rate of lasting success. Removal of calcium from the valve under direct vision with the aid of the pump-oxygenator, along with separation of the leaflets, may reestablish a fair (though not normal) aortic orifice and significantly reduce or even eliminate the obstruction at the valve. However, in many patients calcium reaccumulates within a few years after the operation and aortic stenosis may recur. Recently, with more successful development of artificial aortic valves (the most popular is the Starr–Edwards ball valve, similar to that used for mitral valve replacement), there has been a growing tendency to replace the natural valve with an artificial valve in cases with heavy deposits of calcium. Even total valve replacement cannot be considered a cure of aortic stenosis, and long-range results of these operations still remain to be determined.

Indications for surgical relief of aortic stenosis are based on balancing the risk of operation with an estimate of the patient's health and survival without operation. Here the physician is usually influenced by the unpredictable course of aortic stenosis, referred to above, so that any severe degree of obstruction at the aortic valve is often considered an adequate reason for surgical treatment, even in patients who still appear in good health and are capable of leading normal or almost normal lives.

AORTIC INSUFFICIENCY

Disease of the aortic valve leading to its incompetence and significant regurgitation into the left ventricle may be caused by a variety of conditions. Rheumatic fever may cause scarring and retraction of the three leaflets, thereby making the valve incompetent. Syphilis, once a common cause of aortic insufficiency, but now quite rare, damages the elastic tissue of the aorta, causing enlargement of the aortic orifice, whereby the valve, with intact leaflets, may become too small to cover the orifice. Aortic insufficiency may be caused by congenital malformations of the leaflet. Bacterial endocarditis commonly affects the aortic valve and may destroy sections of it, producing permanent insufficiency after the infection is healed. Aortic insufficiency may be caused by a rupture of a valve from a blow on the chest, or such rupture may occur spontaneously. Aortic insufficiency may also be related to a distortion of the aortic orifice in some forms of dissecting aneurysm of the aorta (see chap. 16) with a normally appearing valve cusp.

As in all other forms of valvular disease, circulatory consequences of aortic insufficiency depend on the extent of valve "involvement." Small amounts of blood regurgitated into the left ventricle are very well tolerated and usually have no significant effect upon the heart and circulation. More severe degrees of aortic insufficiency increase the work load on the left ventricle, in a fashion similar to mitral insufficiency: the left ventricle has to eject not only the quantity of blood destined for the systemic circulation, but also the amount which has regurgitated back into it in diastole. Aortic regurgitation produces a signficantly increased work load on the left ventricle when the amount of blood regurgitated exceeds the amount actually moving forward with each beat. For example, a left ventricular work load is significantly increased when 50 percent of blood ejected regurgitates: in order to maintain a forward flow of 75 cc. of blood with each heart contraction, 150 cc. has to be ejected by the left ventricle, because 75 cc. will regurgitate back into the ventricle during the next diastole. In severe cases of aortic insufficiency, regurgitation may involve as much as 75 percent of left ventricular output; that is, for each liter of blood destined to supply the body, four liters have to be ejected, because three liters will regurgitate back into the ventricle.

Aortic insufficiency has another effect upon the circulation: since the left ventricle ejects such large quantities of blood, the ejection occurs abruptly and the aorta is suddenly distended during systole, but during diastole it empties in two directions equally abruptly. Consequently, the systolic arterial pressure is higher and the diastolic pressure lower than in normal individuals (*wide pulse pressure*) and the pulse acquires a characteristic collapsing quality (*water-hammer pulse*). In the normal individual the blood pressure is 125/80 mm. Hg; in a patient with severe aortic insufficiency it may be 180/40 mm. Hg. Elevated systolic pressure in the latter case does not constitute "high blood pressure" but merely reflects the altered mode of the left ventricular pumping action.

Overloading of the left ventricle leads to considerable dilatation of this heart chamber—left ventricular enlargement—which is much more pronounced than in aortic stenosis. It is noteworthy that significant aortic insufficiency, even with considerable enlargement of the heart, may be well tolerated for many years, even decades, and need not produce disability. Eventually, however, heart failure develops, with its usual chain of events.

The course of aortic insufficiency is less unpredictable than that of aortic stenosis. In the latter sudden death or deterioration, though not common, presents a threat which makes the physician cautious in treating such patients. In aortic insufficiency, on the other hand, such sudden changes are uncommon; deterioration as a rule gives enough warning to physician and patient to allow for a carefully planned course of action. A few patients develop chest pain resembling anginal pain, but its incidence is much smaller than that occurring in aortic stenosis; furthermore, chest pain of aortic insufficiency does not carry the same ominous significance of sudden death which is implied in aortic stenosis accompanied by such pain. The principal complication of aortic insufficiency is subacute bacterial endocarditis, which most frequently affects the aortic valve. It has been stated that residual damage from healed subacute bacterial endocarditis accounts for a certain number of cases of aortic insufficiency. Furthermore, bacterial endocarditis developing on an already insufficient aortic valve almost always accentuates the degree of valve regurgitation, often producing more pronounced enlargement of the heart and its failure.

The diagnosis of aortic insufficiency is relatively easy: not only does the telltale heart murmur indicate incompetence of the aortic valve, but the quality of the arterial pulse and the level of diastolic pressure permit a reasonable estimation of its severity. The size of the heart, furthermore, provides a clue as to the capability of the left ventricle to carry the increased work load.

Treatment of aortic insufficiency may be unnecessary, even if the heart is considerably enlarged. However, when progressive disability develops, surgical treatment is indicated. It almost always involves aortic valve replacement with an artificial prosthesis. Since surgical valve replacement is relatively new, the experience with surgical treatment of aortic insufficiency is still rather limited. Because of the often benign course of this disease on the one hand, and the higher than average risk of the operation and the lack of long-term observations on the other hand, a conservative approach to the selection of cases for surgical treatment is still justified.

TRICUSPID STENOSIS AND
INSUFFICIENCY

Compared with the two heart valves on the left side of the heart (mitral and aortic), diseases of the right-sided valves are rare. Pulmonary stenosis is almost always caused by congenital defects. Tricuspid valve disease may be acquired in two ways: (*a*) as an organic disease, usually caused by rheumatic fever and occurring *in addition* to the involvement of the mitral valve or the mitral and aortic valves. Such rheumatic damage to the tricuspid valve commonly produces a combination of stenosis and insufficiency of that valve. (*b*) Insufficiency of the tricuspid valve may occur with intact valve cusps because of a stretching of the tricuspid orifice, usually related to the failure and dilatation of the right ventricle. This form of tricuspid valve disease— pure insufficiency—is secondary to a variety of diseases of the right side of the heart or of the pulmonary circulation, and is usually referred to as "relative" tricuspid insufficiency. This malfunction of the valve is reversible if treatment improves the performance of the right ventricle.

The effect of tricuspid valve disease upon the circulation is an increased work load upon the right ventricle due to regurgitation through the incompetent valve, analogous to the effects of mitral insufficiency upon the left ventricle. Tricuspid stenosis dams the blood in the right atrium and the great veins entering it. Both stenosis and insufficiency of the tricuspid valve facilitate accumulation of fluid in the tissues (edema), and may result in damage to the liver from severe congestion of that organ. Inasmuch as tricuspid valve disease very rarely occurs without associated mitral valve disease, tricuspid disease is usually "in the shadow" of the more serious lesions of the mitral or aortic valves which produce most of the problems for the patient. Consequently tricuspid disease is usually looked upon as a secondary factor, aggravating already existing problems.

The diagnosis of tricuspid disease is usually quite simple.

Though murmurs, so helpful in the diagnosis of diseases of valves of the left side of the heart, are less constant and reliable, examination and observation of veins (particularly the easily accessible veins in the neck) can usually establish the diagnosis of tricuspid valve disease.

Treatment is often directed toward correction of heart failure; vigorous treatment may completely abolish relative tricuspid insufficiency. Surgical treatment of the tricuspid valve is less well known than that of the other valves. In significant tricuspid stenosis (usually due to fusion of the three leaflets) surgical separation of these leaflets may completely relieve the obstruction. Plastic operations correcting tricuspid insufficiency have been performed in a number of cases, but it is difficult to evaluate their effectiveness, for they have almost always been associated with surgical correction of diseases of other valves. It is usually impossible to estimate how important the additional work on the tricuspid valve was to the over-all results. Recently, in the presence of severe tricuspid insufficiency, artificial valves of the Starr–Edwards ball-valve type have been placed in the tricuspid orifice simultaneously with replacements for other diseased valves, but, here again, evaluation of this additional surgical procedure will have to await some long-term observation; the rationale for such operations has not yet been established.

COMBINED DISEASES OF HEART VALVES

Combined diseases of heart valves include two types: (*a*) combinations of stenosis and insufficiency of the same valve, and (*b*) involvement of more than one valve. In the foregoing discussion stenosis and insufficiency of the mitral and the aortic valves were discussed as separate lesions. This is true for a fair proportion of cases, perhaps more than half. However, in a sizeable number of cases a deformity of one of these two valves affects a valve in such a manner that it becomes obstructed and incompetent at the same time. This is particularly true for scarred valves undergoing calcification in which a valve is in a fixed or semifixed position, being unable either to open or close completely.

Involvement of more than one valve is quite common in a widespread disease of the endocardium, such as rheumatic fever, which frequently affects both the mitral and aortic valves, and occasionally the tricuspid valve as well.

In discussing the four principal lesions of the mitral and aortic valves it was shown that each lesion presents a specific pattern and has its characteristic features, complications, and course. In combined afflictions of heart valves these features are often present in relation to the predominant valve lesion. Thus, a patient may have a combination of mitral stenosis and insufficiency, and aortic insufficiency. While, technically, two valves are incompetent and one of them is too narrow, the physician may assess the situation and find that mitral stenosis is the dominant lesion. In such a case, insufficiency of the two valves may be trivial but the obstruction of the mitral valve highly significant; then the patient follows the course of pure mitral stenosis. In another case, mitral stenosis may be combined with aortic insufficiency, with the latter the predominant lesion, and only mild obstruction at the mitral valve. This patient would then resemble a case of pure aortic insufficiency. There are some cases in which two or three valves are involved, with equal severity and significance, but these are in the minority and probably represent less than 25 percent of the cases of valvular heart disease.

Combined valvular heart disease considerably complicates the diagnosis and the over-all evaluation of a case. It was emphasized earlier that in pure valve lesions the physician can usually make the diagnosis accurately by means of physical diagnosis, X-ray examination, and electrocardiogram. Special tests may be needed to assess the severity of the lesion if surgical treatment is contemplated. In combined valve lesions there may be considerable difficulty in identifying the lesions and, when this has been done, in selecting the predominant from the insignificant lesions. Complicated studies may be necessary, including cardiac catheterization and angiocardiography to evaluate such cases and assess their suitability for surgical treatment.

Treatment of such lesions by surgical means poses great difficulty to the cardiac team, the cardiologist and surgeon alike. Theoretically, it is now possible to replace two or even three valves with artificial prostheses, but the risk of such surgical feats is higher than replacement of a single valve. Considering the fact that in a case of combined valve lesion the solution may lie in correction of only one predominant lesion, without aiming at perfection in correcting all lesions, the judgment to select the lowest-risk operation with the highest possibility of success requires great skill and experience and poses a real challenge to those handling the case.

13

Birth Defects
of the Heart

*The emotional impact of a crippled child is so great that the sub-
ject of congenital diseases of the heart is constantly in the limelight. This attention has been enhanced by the almost miraculous
operations which have been developed in recent years. Surgical
treatment of some forms of congenital cardiac defects presents the
most satisfying results in the entire field of heart disease, for here
a complete and unequivocal cure of a chronic disease is possible.
The experience of seeing a deeply blue child, hardly able to walk
across the room, turning pink after the operation and running
around the hospital corridors within two weeks, is unforgettable
for the parents and the physician alike. And yet, not all parents
are lucky enough to see this happen: some defects are not amenable to surgical treatment at all; others can only be partially corrected. The subject is one of almost infinite complexity, for birth
defects often appear in combinations of two, three, or more together. Nowhere is the diagnostic acumen of the physician more
taxed than in this field; nowhere are decisions so crucial. Such
decisions have to include the need for operation and the time for
operation, as well as the feasibility of surgical correction. This
chapter presents merely the highlights of a complex subject.*

Birth defects affecting the heart and the principal blood vessels
rank among the most common and significant congenital malformations of the body. Interest in congenital heart disease has

been very great in the past two decades. This is due to two reasons: the highly complex subject presents a real challenge to the sophisticated cardiologist-diagnostician; furthermore, correction of some defects by surgical operations has led to some of the most dramatic developments of modern cardiac surgery.

In contrast to other forms of heart disease, congenital heart defects present an almost infinite qualitative variety of conditions afflicting the heart, rather than degrees of progression of a relatively well-defined process. In order to grasp even the crudest concepts of this very complicated subject, it may be helpful to present briefly the progress of the formation and development of the heart.

EMBRYOLOGY OF THE HEART

The heart is formed toward the end of the first month and during the early part of the second month of fetal life. Thus, during the last seven months of pregnancy the heart is fully developed and, except for growth, is almost unchanged up to the time of birth. The formation of the heart begins when a group of cells form a tube, usually referred to as the *primitive cardiac tube,* which is located at the ventral (front) part of the embryo. This hollow tube has two ends, the *venous* end and the *arterial* end. With growth, the tube develops turns, assuming first the shape of the letter U, then the shape of an S. The venous end of the S-shaped loop then bulges out, forming a chamber, which is the primitive single atrium. The middle section of the loop enlarges into the primitive single ventricle. The arterial portion of the tube grows into an arterial trunk. At the end of the first month of pregnancy there is thus a single atrium, a single ventricle, and a single arterial trunk. At the same time, blood vessels begin to grow independently, to join later with the primitive heart. During the early part of the second month of pregnancy, the detailed structures of the heart are formed. Out of two opposite walls of the primitive atrium, cells form ridges growing into a septum, which is completed when the two ridges meet and separate the chamber into two parts. A similar division takes place within the ventricle, which becomes partitioned into two chambers. Between the primitive atrium and ventricle a group of cells form a "cushion" (*endocardial cushion*), which grows into the lower part of the atrial and ventricular septum and forms the mitral and tricuspid valves. Relatively late, a partition is formed within the single trunk, separating it into the pulmonary artery (in front and to the left) and the aorta (in back and to the right). The pulmonary and aortic valves are formed from groups of cells growing out of the lowest portion of the arterial trunk.

While the heart of a two-month old fetus resembles the adult heart, the *function* of the heart develops much later than its structure. Later in the course of pregnancy the wall of the ventricles consolidates its musculature and, when the blood is formed and the entire vascular system is complete, the heart assumes its function as a pump, contracting and relaxing rhythmically as it does after birth. However, the course of the fetal circulation (fig. 27) is entirely different from that after birth.

The principal difference between the fetal circulation and permanent circulation after birth is that the process of oxygenation does not occur in the fetal lungs, for they do not contain air. During the last few months of pregnancy all the tissues of the body are formed and have to be supplied with oxygenated blood in order to survive. The process of oxygenating the blood and of removing the carbon dioxide which has formed in fetal tissues occurs in the placenta, so that the mother's body assumes responsibility for these processes. As shown in figure 27, oxygenated blood returning from the placenta through the umbilical vein enters the inferior vena cava, where it mixes with the blood returning from the fetal lower extremities. The blood in the right atrium of the fetus thus contains a mixture of oxygenated and unoxygenated blood. This mixture is divided into two portions: one enters the pulmonary artery, and the other passes through the *foramen ovale* to the left atrium, and hence to the left ventricle and the aorta. The blood entering the pulmonary artery supplies the lungs, which are contracted and void of air,

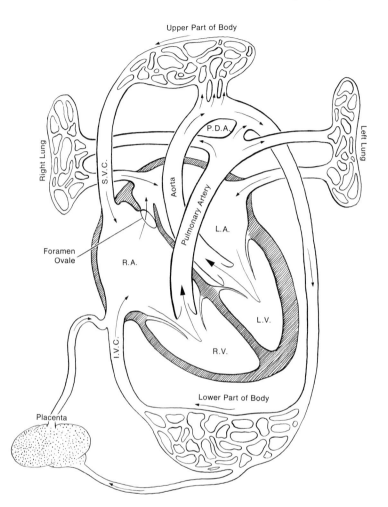

FIGURE 27. *Diagrammatic presentation of the fetal circulation. Description in text. (Abbreviations: R.A., right atrium; R.V., right ventricle; L.A., left atrium; L.V., left ventricle; P.D.A., ductus arteriosus; S.V.C., superior vena cava; I.V.C., inferior vena cava.)*

but most of the blood is directed through the *ductus arteriosus*—a connection between the aorta and the pulmonary artery—into the aorta. Thus it is seen that in the fetal circulation the two sides of the heart are not separated but are joined by two channels not present in the adult: the foramen ovale, an opening between the two atria; and the ductus arteriosus, a large blood vessel connecting the main pulmonary artery with the descending aorta, usually just below the origin of the left subclavian artery. It can also be seen that tissues in the fetus are not supplied by fully oxygenated arterial blood but by a mixture of arterial and venous blood. The head and upper extremities are supplied primarily by this mixed blood entering the left atrium, the left ventricle, and the aorta; the remainder of the body is supplied largely by the blood entering the aorta through the ductus arteriosus. The circulatory course is completed by the umbilical arteries, which connect branches of the lower aorta with the placenta, bringing the mixed blood for reoxygenation.

At the moment of birth, when the infant takes its first breaths, the lungs expand and draw most of the blood from the pulmonary artery into the lungs rather than into the ductus arteriosus. This channel may still function for a few hours but eventually contracts, closes down entirely, and remains in the body as a mere strand of tissue without any opening. Simultaneously, the foramen ovale, which by a valve-like structure permits the blood to flow from right to left, but not in the reverse direction, is held closed by the fall in pressure in the right side of the heart as compared with the left. The foramen ovale then seals itself off entirely in most infants, but this sealing may be incomplete. However, lower pressure in the right atrium than in the left, which persists through life in normal individuals, keeps this opening permanently closed, even if not sealed.

CAUSES OF CONGENITAL DEFECTS

The cause of congenital heart disease is not entirely known. A congenital heart defect falls into one of three categories. It may be a genetically determined hereditary error; it may represent some form of injury during the critical weeks of the formation of the heart; it may, finally, be the result of some disease afflicting the mother (and fetus) during late pregnancy after the heart is fully formed.

The understanding of the hereditary nature of congenital heart disease is still incomplete, although recent developments in genetics and the availability of studies of the chromosomes have clarified some aspects of it. The hereditary occurrence of cardiac defects is manifested by its appearance in more than one member of a family, and by the participation of cardiac defects in well-defined hereditary "syndromes" affecting many organs of the body. Fortunately, hereditary heart defects are a small minority of the cases of congenital heart disease. While exact figures are difficult to compile and are not readily available, it is estimated that the incidence of hereditary types of congenital heart disease is somewhere between 1 and 2 percent. It is some consolation to parents who have the misfortune of having a child with congenital heart disease to know that the chance of having another child with a heart malformation is probably less than 1 in 50, unless other cases of congenital heart disease have occurred in the family.

The types of injury to the fetus during the first two months of pregnancy include, first of all, infection. If the mother develops an infectious illness, particularly one caused by a virus, then there is a strong possibility of malformation of the fetus, especially the heart. The best-known and most completely documented type of infection is German measles, which, if contracted by pregnant women during the critical period, produces a very high percentage of deformed children. Other viral infections in the mother are also suspected of producing such effects upon the fetus, but are not as well proven as German measles. Other forms of injury have been implicated as causes of congenital heart malformation in experimental animals. Among those are: nutritional deficiencies (particularly vitamin deficiencies); reduced oxygen content; drugs; and other agents. There is only indirect evidence that such agents play a part in humans. For example, it has been noted that the incidence of congenital heart disease in children born in high altitudes (above 10,000 feet) is higher than in the general population. The deformity-producing effect of low oxygen tension is here suggested. The famous thalidomide episode did not specifically implicate heart defects, but the fact that serious congenital defects in general may be directly traced to a drug suggests that such a relationship exists.

The possibility of damage to the fetal heart already formed has received less attention in recent years than in the past. The term "fetal endocarditis" suggested a process acquired in the uterus presumably from an illness in the mother, which is analogous to heart diseases later in life (such as rheumatic fever). While this has not been entirely disproved, it is considered an unlikely cause of congenital heart disease, accounting probably for very rare cases.

The *incidence* of congenital heart disease is estimated as somewhere between 0.3 and 0.8 percent of births. Statistics vary widely and are rather inaccurate, since many cases are not discovered until some time after birth, or even later in life, while others may correct themselves spontaneously. Congenital heart disease is the principal form of heart disease in children under the age of four, and a large fraction of such cases in childhood, adolescence, and young adulthood.

The significance of congenital heart disease varies from totally unimportant imperfections associated with a normal life expectancy to such severe deformity of the heart that life is impossible, so that children are stillborn or die within the first few days of life. The number of known defects of the heart and major vessels is great, since deformities of the cardiovascular system occur frequently in more than one area and in a large variety of combinations. However, the vast majority of cases consist of a small number of well-defined defects: ventricular septal defect, atrial septal defect, patent ductus arteriosus, coarctation of the aorta, pulmonary stenosis, aortic stenosis, and transposition of the great vessels.

The effect of the various congenital defects upon the circulation varies greatly, but some of them constitute rather unique situations, affecting the circulatory system differently than do acquired diseases of the heart. The principal effects are due to two basic mechanisms: (*a*) shunting of blood between the two sides of the circulation, and (*b*) obstruction to blood flow.

Shunting of blood between the left and right sides of the heart occurs normally in the fetus (see above) but ceases immediately after birth. Congenital openings (*septal defects*) between chambers provide an opportunity for blood to be shunted after birth. The direction of the shunt depends upon which side has higher pressure and offers more resistance to the flow of blood. The usual direction of flow through shunts is from the greater to the lesser circulation (*left-to-right shunt*); this reflects normal pressure relationship between the two sides. The effect of such left-to-right shunting of blood depends, of course, on the amount shunted; in general, left-to-right shunts result in an increased amount of blood flowing through the lungs. Such shunting, however, has no influence upon blood oxygenation, since fully oxygenated blood returns to the lungs. However, if in addition to a connection between the two sides of the heart, conditions arise which tend to increase pressure within the right side of the heart, then the direction of the shunt reverses and a *right-to-left* shunt develops. Then poorly oxygenated blood returning to the heart for oxygenation will be shunted into the left side and ejected into the aorta without being oxygenated. In the presence of right-to-left shunts blood in the arterial circulation supplying the body will consist of a mixture of fully oxygenated blood returning from the lungs, and poorly oxygenated blood shunted from the right side of the heart. The over-all oxygen saturation of the arterial blood will therefore decrease and may reach the point where blue color of the skin and lips will become apparent ("blue babies"), representing *congenital heart disease with cyanosis*.

Congenital obstruction to the blood flow is due to a narrowing (stenosis) of an orifice at the valve, below the valve, or above the valve. If such stenosis is the only lesion, then it has an effect similar to acquired stenosis of cardiac valves. If however, it is associated with defects in the septum, it may, in addition, alter the course of circulation by reversing the direction of shunt. such obstructions on the right side of the heart are the most important cause of right-to-left shunts and therefore of cyanosis.

THE MORE COMMON MALFORMATIONS

It is obviously impossible to include in the discussion all forms of congenital heart disease. However, the few to be presented in detail constitute more than 90 percent of cases of congenital heart disease. The more important of the rarer lesions will also be briefly defined.

ATRIAL SEPTAL DEFECT

Defects in the atrial septum are related to improper closure of the septum during the period of the formation of the heart. The common variety of this lesion is a defect of the final formation of the septum (a persistence of the "secondary" opening, hence the commonly used term *secundum type* of atrial septal defect). A hole which may be as small as 1 cm. in diameter or as large as most of the atrial septum, is located in the center, the upper, or the posterior part of the atrial septum (fig. 28). It may or may not include the foramen ovale. As a rule, failure of the foramen ovale to close after birth is not equivalent to an atrial septal defect, since it is normally protected by a valve flap, but, in some cases, failure to form the valve flap may be a variant of atrial septal defect. The second type of atrial septal defect is called the *septum primum type* of atrial septal defect. It represents an error in the earlier stage of development, a persistence of a primary opening between the atria which occurs during the early stage of the formation of the septum and then normally closes up. This primal type of defect is located in the lower part of the atrial septum directly adjoining the tricuspid valve. It is often associated with additional malformations involving the tricuspid valve and the mitral valve, either of which may be incompetent, and it is sometimes also accompanied by a defect in the ventricular septum. The primal type of atrial septal defect with its associated abnormalities is related to an improper formation of the *endocardial cushions* during the stage of heart formation and is often referred to as *endocardial cushion defect.*

Regardless of the location and the type of atrial septal defect, its effect upon the circulation depends upon the quantity of blood shunted through it. This in part is related to the size of the defect and in part to the differences in pressure between the two sides. As a rule, large quantities of blood enter the right side of the heart and are ejected into the lungs. Thus the blood returning to the heart from the venae cavae is mixed in the right

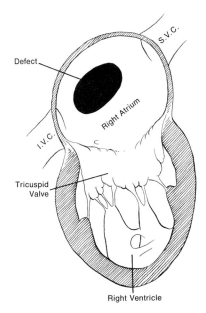

FIGURE 28. *Semidiagrammatic presentation of a typical atrial septal defect. (Abbreviations: I.V.C., inferior vena cava; S.V.C., superior vena cava.)*

atrium with fully oxygenated blood shunted from the left atrium through the defect. In the average case, two, three, or four times as much blood comes from the shunt as from the great veins. Therefore, the pulmonary artery, containing blood destined for the lungs, may show a proportion of only 25 percent from the natural channels and 75 percent from the left side of the heart. As a consequence, blood flow in the pulmonary artery (*pulmonary flow*) is greatly increased. For example, the adult circulation requires at least 5 liters of blood to supply the body. In a normal individual each side of the heart pumps 5 liters per minute. In atrial septal defect body demands are normal, and 5 liters per minute are pumped by the left ventricle into the aorta. However, the right ventricle at the same time pumps 20 liters per minute, 15 liters of which come from the atrial shunt. This large volume of blood entering the lungs increases the work load of the right ventricle, which develops dilatation and hypertrophy, and may eventually fail. As a rule, however, this increased work load of the right ventricle is well tolerated, at least in childhood and adolescence. In spite of considerable enlargement of the heart some individuals live active lives and survive until old age; however, most patients develop significant difficulties in their middle age.

There are two common complications of atrial septal defect: in children, the large blood flow through the lungs appears to be associated with lowered resistance to respiratory infections, and such children may suffer from repeated chest colds and pneumonias. In later years, prolonged overfilling of the pulmonary vessels with blood may result in a rise in pressure in the pulmonary artery. The cause of this is not quite clear, though it may in some way be related to wear and tear of the small pulmonary arterioles from increased blood flow. Such development of pulmonary hypertension occurs in some 25 percent of adults and may have disastrous results. As pressure in the pulmonary artery increases, it is more difficult for blood to enter the lungs and the excessive blood flow through the defect is eventually reduced. Ultimately, so much resistance is offered to flow within the right side of the heart that the shunt becomes reversed (right to left instead of left to right), and the patient develops cyanosis. It is obvious that, as the pressure rises in the pulmonary circulation, the increased work load upon the right ventricle becomes accentuated. Right ventricular overload remains high even if the magnitude of the shunt is reduced or its direction reversed. However, while a large left-to-right shunt of an atrial septal defect with normal pulmonary arterial pressures can be cured by surgical closure of the defect, once pulmonary hypertension arises and the blood flow through the defect declines, the operation is less effective. If the shunt reverses, surgical treatment is no longer possible and the patient sooner or later develops heart failure.

It should be clear from the foregoing discussion that the course of atrial septal defect depends upon the magnitude of the shunt through it and upon the development of its principal complication, pulmonary hypertension. Atrial septal defect can usually be suspected by clinical examination. Even though heart murmurs are neither as characteristic nor as constant in this condition as they are in other forms of congenital heart disease, certain physical findings, the X-ray appearance of the heart shadow, and changes in the electrocardiogram enable the expert to make such a diagnosis. However, the final diagnosis, the magniture of the shunt, and the pulmonary artery pressure are determined by means of cardiac catheterization.

Treatment of atrial septal defect is purely surgical. In childhood, atrial septal defect may appear as a benign lesion, for, except for the children's proneness to respiration infection, their growth and development are usually normal; such children can often indulge in unlimited exercise. However, it is generally believed that surgical closure should be performed before the child is fully grown, in order to protect him from the possible development of pulmonary hypertension.

VENTRICULAR SEPTAL DEFECT

Most defects in the ventricular septum are located in the region of the membranous septum (see chap. 2) and are related to the failure of the lower embryonic septum, growing upward from the ventricular wall, to meet the upper septum, growing down from the arterial trunk. Such a defect is depicted in figure 29. In a small number of cases, ventricular septal defects are located in other areas than the membranous septum and are caused by imperfect formation of the muscular septum. Ventricular septal defects vary from 2 mm. to 3 cm. in diameter. Larger ventricular septal defects are often associated with other malformations of the heart and will be discussed in this connection later; smaller ones are more likely to appear as sole lesions.

The presence of an opening between two pumps performing with entirely different pressures may have profound effect upon their performance. A smaller opening may cause a "leak"—a left-to-right shunt between the two ventricles—but this may not seriously affect the performance of the two pumps. However, when the defect reaches a certain critical size, the two pumps cannot perform separately, but have to eject blood as a joint, single pump. This implies that pressures within the two ventricles have to be identical. It has been shown that the critical

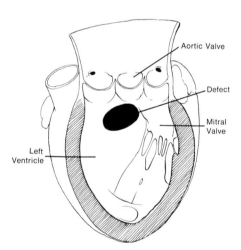

FIGURE 29. *Semidiagrammatic presentation of a typical ventricular septal defect.*

dividing line between those defects which act merely as a path for a simple shunt and those which necessitate an equilibration of pressures in the two chambers is an opening about 1.5 cm. in diameter in the adult heart (children's sizes are correspondingly smaller). Ventricular septal defects associated with such equilibration of pressure are usually referred to as "large" (1.5 to 3 cm. in diameter); those in which the pressure relationship may remain normal are called "small" (less than 1.5 cm. in diameter).

Because of these important circulatory considerations ventricular septal defects differ fundamentally depending upon whether they fall into the category of "small" or "large" ones. Consequently, the two types will be presented separately.

The *small ventricular septal defect* is a congenital lesion which varies in its consequences depending on the size of the opening, and therefore on the size of the shunt. Pressure within the right ventricle usually remains at its normal low level. Blood flowing from a high-pressure left ventricle into the low-pressure right ventricle through a small opening attains high velocity and produces very loud murmurs. The intensity of such murmurs is not necessarily related to the magnitude of the shunt; as a matter of fact, some of the loudest murmurs are produced by the smallest ventricular septal defects. Defects in this category are considered "small" from the standpoint of the pressure relationships between the two ventricles; they can, however, be associated with fairly large left-to-right shunts. The effect of such defects upon the circulation, and their corresponding seriousness, is largely the function of the magnitude of the shunts. It is customary to subdivide such ventricular septal defects into two groups: those with shunts small enough not to disturb normal circulatory dynamics, and those with larger shunts which produce significant "strain" upon the heart.

Ventricular septal defects associated with shunts of less than 50 percent of the output of the left ventricle alter the circulation very little. Except for the loud murmurs, patients afflicted with such ventricular septal defects have no symptoms, their heart is not enlarged, and their X-ray examinations and electrocardiogram are usually normal. It is assumed that such patients have an almost normal life expectancy, and the only significant danger is the possibility of subacute bacterial endocarditis in the region of the defect. Such small defects have been known to close off spontaneously, but the incidence of such spontaneous cures is not yet known and is probably rather rare. Such a small ventricular septal defect, associated with normal findings except for a murmur, is often referred to as "Roger's disease."

Ventricular septal defects associated with left-to-right shunts larger than 50 percent of the left ventricular output and showing normal pressures within the right side of the heart may present a much more serious picture than the preceding group. Such shunts may be two or three times as large as the left ventricular output, in which case the large shunt will increase flow to the lung in a manner similar to the atrial septal defect. Such patients often develop cardiac enlargement and abnormalities in the X ray and electrocardiogram; they may become disabled by symptoms and may proceed into heart failure.

It is obvious from the foregoing discussion that the "small" ventricular septal defect really presents a wide range of conditions varying from innocent to serious heart lesions. The physician can usually make the diagnosis by physical examination and the simpler auxiliary diagnostic procedures. However, only cardiac catheterization can demonstrate the magnitude of the shunt and the resulting derangement of the circulation.

The treatment of the small ventricular septal defect consists of its surgical closure with the aid of the pump-oxygenator. The indications for such surgical treatment depend upon the effect of the defect on the circulation. It is generally believed that, if the shunt is small, such an operation should not be recommended because the outlook of untreated patients is so good that even the modest risk of an operation is not justified. On the other hand, if the shunt is large, surgical correction is urgently needed to avoid problems in the future. There is no general agreement as to where the dividing line is between the two categories. In most cardiac centers, shunts greater than twice the left ventricular output are considered suitable for closure; those less than 50 percent of left ventricular output are usually left alone. In the intermediate group individual decisions are made.

While the category of "small" ventricular defects presents a mixture of innocent and significant lesions, *large ventricular septal defects* are always serious. Their essential feature is severe pulmonary hypertension, present since birth. The reader will recall from chapter 3 that the normal systolic pressure in the right ventricle and in the pulmonary artery is about 25 mm. Hg, while that in the left ventricle and the aorta is 120 mm. Hg. If the large communication between the ventricles causes an increase in pressure in the right ventricle to a level identical with that in the left, then pressures in the right ventricle and the pulmonary artery have to rise to a level approximately five times that of normal. Such pressure can only be maintained in one of two ways: either the arterioles in the lungs constrict and produce high resistance, or the blood flow to the lungs becomes very large. The general subject of pulmonary hypertension will be discussed in more detail in chapter 15.

Thus, an infant born with a "large" ventricular septal defect will survive only if a large volume of blood can be accommodated in the lungs or if his pulmonary arterioles are capable of constricting. The *high-flow* and *high-resistance* types of pulmonary hypertension set a pattern shortly after birth which often persists for a lifetime.

The *high-flow* ventricular septal defect may cause serious difficulties during the first year of life. Even though the shunt is purely left to right, so that infants do not show cyanosis, such infants often develop respiratory distress, excessive cardiac enlargement, and heart failure. A certain number of infants may face death, and, in order to save their lives, it may be necessary to perform a palliative surgical operation consisting of placing a constricting band around the main pulmonary artery (*banding operation*), which reduces the flow to the lungs without lowering the pressure in the right ventricle. The first year of life is a critical period, but afterwards children improve and may grow and develop normally. Some children are considerably limited in their activities, but others do surprisingly well and have an almost normal tolerance for effort.

The most important feature of the high-flow type of pulmonary hypertension associated with large ventricular septal defect is the fact that the elevated pressure in the pulmonary artery is maintained exclusively or largely by the high flow. It follows that if the ventricular septal defect were closed, so that the shunt and the resulting high flow would cease, then pressure in the pulmonary circulation might return to normal. Thus, an operation has a beneficial effect.

The large ventricular septal defects associated with *high-resistance* pulmonary hypertension may be better tolerated in infancy. Cardiac enlargement is less pronounced and may even be absent. Shortness of breath and heart failure are rare. However, the cardinal feature of such cases is that the resistance in the pulmonary circulation may approach or even exceed the resistance in the greater circulation. In the presence of such high pulmonary resistance the flow through the defect may be either from left to right or from right to left, depending upon which of the two outlets offers less resistance to flow. Thus, pulmonary hypertension may be so high at birth that the direction of the shunt through the septal defect is reversed, producing blueness (cyanosis). In other cases, such reversal of shunt with cyanosis may develop gradually some time during life. This type of large ventricular septal defect combined with cyanosis is referred to as the "Eisenmenger complex," at one time thought to be a specific form of congenital heart disease but now merely considered a variant of large ventricular septal defect.

In contrast to the high-flow type, the high-resistance type of large ventricular septal defects is not amendable to surgical treatment. Patients with right-to-left shunts not only are not helped if the septal defect is closed but may get worse. Those who still have left-to-right shunts are occasionally operated upon, but the results are seldom worthwhile; the principal objective of the operation—reduction of pressure in the pulmonary circulation—cannot be met except in a minor way.

The course of the large ventricular septal defect is variable. The serious difficulty that may occur in infancy has already been mentioned. Patients who are inoperable may survive into middle life. Occasionally such patients live to be 50 or 60, but these are exceptions. The principal concern in the problem of the large ventricular septal defect is the possibility that some patients belonging in the operable high-flow type may change into the inoperable high-resistance type. Such transition occurs in adults and in older children; whether it occurs during the first ten years of life remains a matter of controversy. In most cardiac centers, children with high-flow ventricular septal defects are operated upon early, before the age of six, in order to avert such a possibility.

Surgical treatment of large ventricular septal defects is performed with the aid of the pump-oxygenator. While the risk of such operations is higher than that for small defects, improvements in technique have brought the risk in most cardiac centers down to reasonable figures. The problem of selecting cases for surgical treatment is the opposite of that involved in small ventricular septal defects. In the latter, patients who need surgical treatment must be separated from those whose lesion is too innocent to undertake the risk of surgery. In large ventricular septal defects, patients who can be helped by the operation must be separated from those who are inoperable. Curiously enough the magnitude of the left-to-right shunt is a decisive factor in both groups, and the same ratio of pulmonary flow to systemic flow (1.5 to 2.0) separates operable cases from innocent ones in one group, and from inoperable ones in the other group.

Summarizing the complex subject of ventricular septal defects, one can distinguish two major groups, with each subdivided further into two types. The "small" ventricular septal defect is characterized by normal or near-normal pressures in the pulmonary artery. Such defects may be small enough to present no significant problems for the patient and require no treatment. Larger defects in this category are amenable to successful surgical treatment with excellent results, often with complete cures.

"Large" ventricular septal defects are associated with severe pulmonary hypertension and often present very serious problems. Within this category there are cases with "high-flow" pulmonary hypertension, which are still amenable to successful surgical treatment; other cases, representing "high-resistance" pulmonary hypertension, are inoperable.

TETRALOGY OF FALLOT

This congenital malformation is one of the many in which a "large" ventricular septal defect plays an essential role. Described originally as a malformation consisting of four abnormalities, it is now considered simply a combination of a large ventricular septal defect with pulmonary stenosis. The term "tetralogy," implying four deviations from the norm, is of mere historical interest, but has established itself so widely that it continues to be used.

The defect in the ventricular septum in tetralogy of Fallot is identical in location and origin with the "large" defect already discussed. The obstruction to the outflow of blood from the right ventricle into the pulmonary artery may occur either at the pulmonary valve or underneath it. The first type (*valvular pulmonary stenosis*) is rarer than the second (*infundibular stenosis*). The physiological effects of tetralogy of Fallot are very similar to those of large ventricular septal defects without pulmonary stenosis. In both, a large connection between the two ventricles equilibrates pressures in these chambers. In both there is a competition between the resistance to outflow into one or the other outlet, which determines in which direction more blood will flow. However, in the plain ventricular septal defect right-sided resistance is located in the pulmonary vascular tree; in tetralogy of Fallot it is located in the right heart itself. Pressure beyond the obstruction is normal, so that blood flows into the lungs under the customary low pressure, in direct contrast with large ventricular septal defect.

The over-all picture of tetralogy of Fallot and its course depends largely upon the degree of obstruction within the outflow tract of the right heart. If the resistance offered by this obstruction is lower than that within the systemic circulation, then left-to-right shunt through the defect will occur. If the obstruction is equal to the systemic, then shunts will be "balanced" or nil. If the obstruction is severe and its resistance higher than in the systemic circulation, then blood will flow from right to left and the patient will be cyanotic. This last variety, the cyanotic form of tetralogy of Fallot, is a common congenital malformation which produces "blue babies." Except for the cyanosis, the effects of tetralogy of Fallot upon the circulation are somewhat less serious than in the uncomplicated ventricular septal defect, since in the former pulmonary hypertension is absent. The high ventricular pressure in the right side of the heart seems to be better tolerated when combined with a ventricular septal defect than when present alone (see pulmonary stenosis, below).

Cyanosis in tetralogy of Fallot shows wide variation, from an almost inconspicuous bluish tinge visible only during crying or exercise to a deep purple color of the entire body. The cyanosis is due to mixing of blood returning from the lungs with the shunted blood bypassing the lungs, and its depth is related to the amount of blood which can reach the lungs for oxygenation. The ratio of blue and pink bloods mixing in the arterial system and providing the color of the skin can undergo change, either in response to exercise, crying, breath holding, or spontaneously, without obvious cause. Such sudden changes producing deeper cyanosis occur in patients with tetralogy of Fallot, particularly in young children, in the form of attacks of cyanosis ("blue spells") which may, under certain circumstances, constitute a threat to life and therefore are considered ominous, often suggesting the need for surgical intervention.

Thus, the principal difference between the large ventricular septal defect alone and such a defect with obstruction to the outflow of blood from the right ventricle (tetralogy of Fallot) is that in the former, heart failure and overfilled pulmonary circulation are the cause of deterioration of the patient, while in the latter, cyanosis and its consequences are in the foreground. Cyanosis, in addition to causing blue color, tiredness, and some shortness of breath (which may make children "squat" when they tire), leads also to an increased number of red blood cells, which makes the blood "thicker" and more difficult to perfuse organs of the body, and enhances clot formation. These factors led to the development of operations which do not correct the malformation of the heart but increase the saturation of arterial blood with oxygen, therefore relieving or completely removing cyanosis and its consequences. The first such operation was the Blalock–Taussig procedure, which consists of creating a connection between a large systemic artery (usually the subclavian) and the pulmonary artery. This connection brings blood from the systemic circulation back to the lung via this "detour," thereby permitting more blood to become oxygenated in the lungs and changing the ratio of the blood mixture in the left heart so that more "pink" and less "blue" blood will be provided for the body. Other operations using similar principles have also been designed and are still used, but they are usually interim procedures in children too small for open-heart surgery in order to give temporary improvement until the complete correction can be performed.

Open-heart surgery for total correction of tetralogy of Fallot is generally considered the treatment of choice. Such operations are possible in most but not all cases, for in some the pulmonary artery beyond the obstruction is so small that, even when the obstruction is relieved, the blood cannot be channeled into the lungs. Because of such variations it is usually necessary to study such patients by cardiac catheterization and also to outline details of the architecture of the heart and the vessels by selective angiocardiography. Such knowledge helps the surgeon to study modes of surgical treatment in advance of the operation.

PULMONARY STENOSIS

Of the four heart valves, the pulmonary valve is the one which, if diseased, is almost always affected from birth and not by processes acquired during life. *Pulmonary stenosis* implies, in common usage, obstruction of blood flow between the right ventricle and the pulmonary artery, regardless of whether this obstruction is in the valve itself, underneath the valve, or, rarely, above the valve. Obstruction within the right ventricle below the valve is usually associated with other malformation, the most common of which is the ventricular septal defect (the two together constitute tetralogy of Fallot; see above). On the other hand, obstruction at the valve is more often an isolated lesion. This difference is explained by the fact that isolated pulmonary stenosis (valvular) is due to an error of fetal development occurring later in the stage of formation of the heart when the septum is already closed.

Valvular pulmonary stenosis is most often caused by congenital fusion (growing together) of the three valve leaflets, which then assume a domelike shape with a small opening in the center. The degree of the obstruction to flow varies from insignificant to very severe. As in stenosis of the aortic valve (described in chap. 12) the pressure is elevated in the ventricle and remains normal in the pulmonary artery. The difference (*pressure gradient*) between the two provides an index of the degree of obstruction. The pulmonary stenosis may be so severe that pressure in the right ventricle is higher than that in the left.

In a certain number of cases of severe valvular pulmonary stenosis, the foramen ovale in newborn babies fails to close. This is understandable, for the very high pressure in the right ventricle elevates pressure in the right atrium as well, whereby the blood flow through the foramen (from right to left) in the fetal circulation continues after birth. In such cases significant amounts of blood can flow through this shunt from right to left to produce lower arterial oxygen saturation and cyanosis.

However, most cases of valvular pulmonary stenosis are not cyanotic, and the effect of the obstruction upon the circulation is to produce overloading of the right ventricle, which eventually may lead to failure of that chamber. In milder cases such overloading of the right circulation may be reasonably well tolerated, but in severe degrees of obstruction activities may be markedly limited in early adult life. The cyanotic form of pulmonary stenosis (pulmonary stenosis with patent foramen ovale) carries an even more ominous outlook. Severe pulmonary stenosis may produce serious trouble, even death, in early infancy. As in ventricular septal defect (see above) a critical period often exists during the first six months of life, which, when passed, may be followed by relatively good growth and development. Pulmonary stenosis is a particularly treacherous lesion in infancy and, since it can be corrected surgically, should be diagnosed early in life.

The diagnosis of pulmonary stenosis can usually be made by a combination of physical examination, X-ray films, and electro-cardiography. Its measurement, and therefore its consideration for surgical treatment, requires the performance of cardiac catheterization. Surgery consists of cutting through the obstructed valve, relieving the obstruction underneath the valve, if there is any, and closing the patent foramen ovale, if present. This operation is not a curative one, for the valve remains deformed, but it is usually possible to reduce the pressure gradient to a totally insignificant one or to abolish it altogether. The valve may become incompetent after the operation, but regurgitation through an incompetent pulmonary valve appears to have little significant adverse effects upon the heart, in contrast to other valves.

PATENT DUCTUS ARTERIOSUS

Technically, patent ductus arteriosus is not a congenital heart lesion, because all infants are born with the ductus arteriosus open. This defect merely represents failure of this fetal channel to close after birth. However, its failure to close is not necessarily related to circumstances existing after birth, for patent ductus arteriosus is a common defect in children born to mothers who had German measles early in pregnancy. As described earlier, the duct connects the first portion of the descending aorta with the main pulmonary artery (see fig. 27). As a result of the failure of this duct to close, a shunt develops between the aorta and the pulmonary artery, the size of which depends upon the size of the duct. Under normal circumstances the presence of patent ductus arteriosus does not influence the normal pressure relationship between the two sides of the heart; therefore, a left-to-right shunt is present, feeding blood from the high-pressure aorta to the low-pressure pulmonary artery. A small duct may have very little influence on the circulation of blood. As in shunts between the two sides of the heart, a shunt through a duct will affect the circulation insignificantly if less than 50 perecent of the blood ejected into the aorta returns to the pulmonary artery. However, patent ductus arteriosus frequently involves a large vessel which is capable of shunting large quantities of blood, so that blood escaping into the pulmonary circulation may be twice the amount of blood supplying the body, or more. As a specific example, if 5 liters of blood per minute is needed to supply the body, the left ventricle has to eject 15 liters per minute because 10 liters return to the lungs. It is obvious that in a large patent ductus arteriosus the *left* ventricle alone is overloaded, for the right ventricle ejects the normal amount of blood (five liters in the example quoted) and is not subjected to high pressure. As a consequence, large patent ductus leads to hypertrophy and dilatation of the left ventricle and, eventually, to left ventricular failure.

Large patent ductus arteriosus may cause serious difficulties during the first few months of life, when heart failure may ensue and lead to death unless recognized and surgically treated. In survivors of this critical period the situation improves during the second year of life, and children may develop normally and lead active lives until early or middle adulthood.

The course of patent ductus arteriosus may be altered by complications, the most important being the development of pulmonary hypertension. In some cases pulmonary hypertension producing pressures in the pulmonary artery equal to those in the aorta may be present at birth or shortly afterwards; in others pressure in the pulmonary artery may increase later in life. The development of pulmonary hypertension has two important consequences: (*a*) it overloads the right ventricle and may lead to its failure; and (*b*) it may gradually eliminate the left-to-right shunt through the duct and replace it with a right-to-left shunt, in which resistance in the pulmonary circulation exceeds that in the systemic circulation. In such cases unoxygenated blood enters the descending aorta and mixes with arterial blood supplying the abdomen and the lower extremities, causing cyanosis only in the legs but not in the head and arms. The other significant complication is the development of bacterial endocarditis, which is relatively common with this condition.

Patent ductus arteriosus was the first congenital defect amenable to surgery. Located outside the heart, the duct can be surgically closed without the need for special equipment or the heart–lung machine. While the operation requires skill and experience, in many medical centers the risk of the operation has been brought down to the very low figure of less than 0.5 percent. Because of its relative safety in many cardiac centers, surgery is performed even when the duct is so small that any permanent effect upon the circulation is unlikely. This is done to prevent bacterial endocarditis, which does not develop after closure of the duct. The main concern in selecting cases for surgical treatment is not the very small but the large duct with pulmonary hypertension. Cases with reversal of blood flow (right-to-left shunt) are inoperable. Those with severe pulmonary hypertension and a small left-to-right shunt are on the borderline of operability: as in ventricular septal defect, once pulmonary hypertension is established without the contribution of a large flow through the lungs, the closure of communication between the two sides of the circulation misses the point and becomes purposeless or even harmful. The possibility that pulmonary hypertension may develop in patients with moderately large or large ducts is a real one, and justifies surgery early in childhood, from the third year of life on.

COARCTATION OF THE AORTA

This malformation affects the aorta rather than the heart, but is usually included under the heading of "congenital heart disease." It consists of a narrowing (often bordering on complete closure) of the descending aorta beyond the exit of the left subclavian artery, at the point where in the fetus the ductus arteriosus enters the aorta (see fig. 27). As a consequence of this malformation blood reaches the abdomen and the lower extremities via "detours," collateral vessels, usually running between the ribs and connecting with the aorta below the point of obstruction. The narrowing of the aorta produces high blood pressure in the arms and head but low blood pressure in the lower part of the body (see chap. 11), and is the most important practical consequence of this malformation. Thus, children with coarctation of the aorta may have hypertension from infancy. In some of them the overloading of the left side of the heart by the elevated arterial blood pressure leads to heart failure, necessitating an operation during the first few months of life. More often, however, coarctation is not recognized until later in life. Sometimes the first abnormal finding is that of high blood pressure.

Diagnosis of coarctation of the aorta can be made on physical examination when higher blood pressure is detected in the arms than in the legs. This diagnosis is supplemented by X-ray examination, and special techniques are seldom necessary. Surgical treatment of coarctation consists of resectioning the narrowed portion and resuturing the two ends of the aorta to each other. Rarely, a synthetic graft may be necessary to connect the two ends. Surgery is indicated whenever there is significant elevation of pressure in the arms.

AORTIC STENOSIS

Congenital aortic stenosis is in many respects similar to acquired aortic stenosis; in fact, it may be related to the acquired form more often than we used to think. The commonest form of congenital aortic stenosis affects the valve, producing either fusion of the three leaflets or fusion of a congenital *bicuspid* valve. A developmental error, producing two rather than three aortic valve cusps, is common. In some cases it may narrow the orifice; in others it may be the basis on which later in life calcium is deposited and calcific aortic stenosis of the adult type develops. The next most common form of aortic stenosis is obstruction underneath the valve, usually consisting of a membrane spread beneath the aortic valve, with an opening in its center. The rarest form of congenital aortic stenosis is a narrowing of the aorta just above the origin of the coronary arteries.

The effects of aortic obstruction upon the circulation have been discussed in connection with acquired valve diseases. The course and treatment of congenital aortic stenosis are analogous to those of acquired disease of this valve. However, severe obstruction of the aortic orifice after birth may cause heart failure in infants. Early recognition and operation in infancy may be lifesaving.

TRANSPOSITION OF GREAT VESSELS

"Transposition" is one of the commoner congenital heart lesions; however, the seriousness of the derangement of circulation resulting from it causes most of the infants thus afflicted to die at birth or shortly after. Some children with transposition do survive beyond the first year of life, but survival to adult life is rare.

The term "transposition" of the arterial trunks signifies a developmental error in which the division of the primitive trunk proceeds in an abnormal fashion so that the aorta is located in front of the pulmonary artery rather than the other way around. The fate of an infant thus afflicted depends upon the association of other abnormalities, which, under certain circumstances, can lessen deformity caused by such malrotation. Consequently, "transposition" is not really a well-defined congenital entity, such as the ones described above, but represents a great number of possible combinations of defects. The complexity of this group of malformations is so great that we can include here only a few comments related to it. There are three principal types of transposition:

Complete transposition of great vessels (see fig. 30). This is the most serious form of transposition. The aorta, located anteriorly, meets with the right ventricle, and the pulmonary artery, located posteriorly, originates from the left ventricle. It is obvious that a newborn with this anomaly cannot survive unless some mitigating circumstances exist. When after birth the normal circulation is established, such an infant has blood returning from the lungs to the left side of the heart pumped back into the lungs through the misplaced pulmonary artery, while the "blue" blood returning from the body is pumped back into the aorta without being oxygenated. Survival in such cases is possible, however, and depends upon the presence of large shunts between chambers. Thus an atrial septal defect with a left-to-right shunt, a ventricular septal defect with such a shunt, and a patent ductus arteriosus, each alone or in combination, may supply *some* oxygenated blood to be mixed with the "blue" blood before being pumped into the aorta. As a rule, the cyanosis in such cases is very intense, but surprisingly enough an occasional patient with complete transposition survives into adult age.

In addition to defects permitting blood shunting, upon which survival depends, complete transposition is often associated with other lesions, such as pulmonary or aortic stenosis, complete absence of one of the cardiac septums, or coarctation of the aorta. In many cases the situation is so complex that a definitive diagnosis is very difficult even with the most sophisticated laboratory tests.

Treatment of complete transposition depends entirely upon the feasibility of partial surgical correction. Complete correction

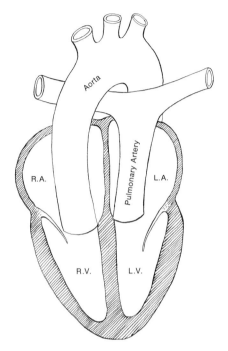

FIGURE 30. *Semidiagrammatic presentation of the circulation in complete
transposition of the great vessels. Communications between the two sides of
the circulation necessary for survival
are not shown in the drawing.*

of this complicated set of lesions is probably beyond realistic
hope, even in the distant future; however, several attempts at
providing more oxygenated blood for the aorta and more "blue"
blood for the pulmonary artery by means of various surgical
measures have been made, some of which have been successful.
The main difficulty is that most of the patients die in infancy
before such surgery can be contemplated.

Partial transposition. Here the arterial trunks are transposed
in a manner similar to complete transposition, but the cardiac

chambers are so located that the circulation is not totally reversed. The two types of partial transposition include: (*a*) cases in which the aorta and the pulmonary artery both originate from the right ventricle, and (*b*) those in which the aorta originates from the right ventricle and the pulmonary artery originates from *both* ventricles (straddling a defect between the two ventricles). Then the circulation of blood depends upon the presence of defects, mostly ventricular septal defect. In such cases not only does blood mixing produce circumstances permitting easy survival, but occasionally the cyanosis is surprisingly mild. This group of malformations is less serious than complete transposition, but still constitutes hazard to life and usually defies total surgical correction.

Corrected transposition. In corrected transposition the abnormal position of the great vessels is identical with that in complete transposition. However, the chambers are also malrotated, to the extent that the anteriorly located aorta meets the left ventricle, while the posteriorly located pulmonary artery meets the right ventricle. Consequently, the heart looks abnormal but the circulation of blood proceeds along the normal pathways. Theoretically, patients who have corrected transposition may have healthy hearts; in practice, however, such malrotation of the heart is almost always associated with some other abnormality. Among the common malformations associated with corrected transposition is a ventricular septal defect, sometimes associated with pulmonary stenosis (tetralogy of Fallot), and a deformity of the mitral valve producing mitral insufficiency. The course and outlook in cases of corrected transposition is entirely that of the associated lesion. Surgical correction is possible in attacking the lesion (not the transposed chambers and trunks) in the same manner as similar lesions without corrected transposition. However, the abnormally located heart chambers may present some technical difficulties to the surgeon, who would consider such cases as having higher risks than identical cases without the transposition.

OTHER MALFORMATIONS OF THE HEART

In the preceding paragraphs eight congenital heart lesions have been discussed. They constitute the bulk of cases of congenital heart disease—more than 90 percent. It has been pointed out that in each of them there are variants and subdivisions. Furthermore, a combination of lesions is quite common: atrial septal defect may be associated with ventricular septal defect or with patent ductus arteriosus. Patent ductus occurs in association with coarctation of the aorta or with ventricular septal defect, and so on. In addition to these principal birth defects of the heart and their combinations, there are a number of other well-defined malformations which deserve brief comment.

Pulmonary atresia. In this condition the outflow tract from the right ventricle is totally closed. The pulmonary artery is diminutive and has no communication with the right ventricle. In such cases there is a large ventricular septal defect through which all the blood from the right side enters the aorta. Circulation to the lungs takes place via collateral arteries originating from some branches of the aorta and through a patent ductus connecting with the pulmonary artery. This condition is very serious, and children seldom survive beyond the first few years. No known treatment is available.

Tricuspid atresia. Here the tricuspid valve is entirely closed and the circulation is rerouted through a large atrial septal defect and a ventricular septal defect. Thus, blood returning to the right side of the heart enters the left atrium through the atrial defect, where it mixes with the fully oxygenated blood. The mixture then enters the left ventricle, where part of it is propelled into the aorta and part enters the right ventricle and hence the pulmonary artery through a ventricular septal defect. In tricuspid atresia the fraction of blood entering the lungs is small, as a rule, and children, deeply cyanotic, may benefit from the Blalock–Taussig operation, which acts here in the same manner as in tetralogy of Fallot. Total correction is not possible. The prognosis is poor with only occasional survival beyond a few years.

Persistent truncus arteriosus. When the primitive arterial trunk fails to divide before birth, a child can be born with a single trunk instead of the two main arteries. In such cases there is a large ventricular septal defect which the large vessel straddles, collecting all the blood from both ventricles. This trunk gives up two branches entering the lungs as pulmonary arteries and then takes the usual course of the aorta.

The course and prognosis in this condition is variable, depending on the amount of blood supplied to the lungs. A good many children die in infancy or early childhood, but some may survive into adulthood or even middle age. There is no known surgical treatment of this malformation.

Ebstein's anomaly. This is a congenital deformity and downward displacement of the tricuspid valve, which is associated with an atrial septal defect. The tricuspid valve is incompetent and the right ventricle is usually weak, so that a portion of blood returning to the right heart enters the left atrium through the atrial septal defect, producing cyanosis. There are various gradations of this deformity, which may be very serious with poor chance of survival beyond infancy, though other patients live well into middle age and lead a reasonably normal life. In more serious cases some attempts have been made to improve the situation by a bypass operation, with variable results.

Single ventricle. It has been stated in connection with ventricular septal defect that even in "large" ventricular septal defects only a small portion of the ventricular septum is missing, with the diameter of the hole no greater than 3 cm. However, in rare cases the entire ventricular septum may be missing, in which case the heart has only a single ventricle. This is one of the more complicated malformations, and almost always other abnormalities are present as well, such as pulmonary or aortic stenosis, or transposition of the arterial trunks. Survival depends upon the combination of the abnormalities, some of which may be more favorable than others. There are cases reported of survival into middle adult life.

Anomalous pulmonary veins. The four pulmonary veins

normally enter the posterior portion of the left atrium. In the presence of congenital heart disease some of the pulmonary veins may be transposed and enter the right instead of the left atrium, particularly if an atrial septal defect exists. This additional malformation is considered a relatively unimportant factor in atrial septal defects, and during the corrective operation the veins can usually be rechanneled into the left atrium.

In contrast to "partial" anomalous pulmonary venous return, there is also a *complete* transposition of the pulmonary veins, in which none of the veins enters the left side of the heart. In this condition, termed *total anomalous pulmonary venous return,* all pulmonary veins empty into an intermediary venous vessel which connects with the *right* atrium. In the commonest course of this malformation, the pulmonary veins empty into a saclike structure directly behind the heart, which connects with the superior vena cava. In this condition survival depends upon the presence of a large atrial septal defect. The blood returning to the right heart contains a mixture of blood from the systemic circulation and the pulmonary circulation. This mixture is divided in the right atrium into the portion which proceeds along the normal pathways and the portion which enters the left atrium and then the left ventricle and aorta.

Anomalous pulmonary venous return has a variety of degrees as far as the cyanosis, course, and prognosis are concerned. In some cases it may lead to failure and early death; in others it permits normal development and relatively symptom-free life as an adult. This condition may be totally correctable by surgery, depending on the course the transposed veins take and the associated lesions.

Mitral valve disease. Congenital mitral valve disease is rare. If present, a deformity of the valve producing regurgitation is found more often than is mitral stenosis. The consequences of mitral valve disease upon the circulation and their treatment are similar to those of acquired mitral disease.

14

Chronic Diseases
of the Heart

Atherosclerosis, hypertension, valvular heart disease, and con-
genital heart disease—discussed in the last four chapters—con-
stitute the "big four" of heart disease. A number of less common
chronic afflictions of the heart will be discussed in this chapter.
These diseases have no relationship to each other and are placed
together here as a "miscellaneous" group simply because they
constitute lesser problems in comparison with those already dis-
cussed and would not justify a special chapter for each.

CHRONIC MYOCARDIAL DISEASES

It has been explained in previous chapters that the consequences
of impaired function of the myocardium are twofold: enlargement of the heart (the earlier stage) and cardiac failure (the
later stage). Malfunction of the heart muscle occurs as a result
of increased work load or of its partial destruction. Both these
mechanisms occupied a prominent place in the preceding four
chapters. If a patient has either enlargement of the heart or heart
failure, the physician logically looks for the four common causes
for these disturbances. When all of them have been excluded, he
then considers other forms of myocardial disease.

In some cases of chronic myocardial disease its mechanism is
known and understood; in others the cause is suspected but not
definitely established; and in still others there is no apparent

cause. In general, chronic myocardial disease is less well known than most of the other forms of heart disease; its classification is blurred and the course of the disease uncertain. Chronic myocardial disease can be subdivided in the following groups:

CHRONIC MYOCARDITIS

In the discussion of acute myocarditis (chap. 9), it was stated that acute inflammatory disease of the heart muscle occurs occasionally in connection with viral or bacterial infections. Acute involvement of the myocardium may lead to death or to recovery, but occasionally results in a chronic, smoldering inflammatory disease of the myocardium—chronic myocarditis. While chronic myocarditis may be a residual disease from acute infectious processes, more often it is an inflammatory disease without an obvious acute stage and usually without a known causative agent. Thus, chronic myocarditis most often develops as a gradual enlargement of the heart associated with a decrease in the patient's capabilities to perform work, and it eventually leads to frank heart failure. The course of chronic myocarditis is variable: sometimes there is an unrelenting downhill progress which cannot be altered by treatment and which leads to death within a matter of months; in other cases the process may be more gradual, may be stopped or delayed by medical treatment, and may last several years. The diagnosis can only be suspected during life, as there are no specific tests which would identify the inflammatory process in the heart and separate it from other chronic myocardial diseases. The ultimate proof of chronic myocarditis depends on the demonstration of inflammatory changes at autopsy.

NUTRITIONAL AND TOXIC HEART DISEASE

In various tropical countries nutritional heart disease plays an important role as a cause of death. In some forms, such as *beriberi heart disease,* the cause is known (vitamin B deficiency); in others, such as the African form of myocardial failure, the specific agent has not been identified. Nutritional heart disease is seldom seen in our civilization with the exception of beriberi heart disease occurring in alcoholics. There is still a controversy whether heart disease found occasionally in chronic alcoholics is a form of nutritional deficiency (due to inadequate intake, poor absorption, or poor utilization of Vitamin B or related compounds) or is, at least in part, due to the direct toxic myocardial damage produced by the alcohol. In early stages of the beriberi type of myocardial disease, the destructive process may be reversed by proper treatment. When established for a long time, the disease is usually irreversible.

Other forms of chronic myocardial disease include a variety of conditions: cardiac enlargement, myocardial weakness, and failure have been found in cases with some generalized systemic disorder, such as sarcoidosis, systemic lupus erythematosus, periarteritis, scleroderma, and so on. Metabolic disorders, such as amyloidosis and glycogen storage disease, affect the myocardium. Furthermore, various forms of generalized diseases of the skeletal muscle may affect the heart muscle as well, such as the various forms of muscular dystrophies and Friedreich's ataxia.

TUMORS OF THE HEART

The heart is one of the organs in the body which is seldom affected by either benign or malignant tumors. In terminal cases of cancer, particularly in cancer of the lungs, malignant cells occasionally invade the heart. However, such growths seldom play a significant role as a form of heart disease, since patients usually die of cancer before heart failure develops, and if it does, the picture is all too clear.

Somewhat more important are malignant diseases of the blood–lymphatic system, such as leukemia and lymphoma. In such cases the heart and the pericardium may be invaded by malignant cells, producing a confusing picture of heart disease while the primary disease may not be apparent.

Rare tumors originating in the heart muscle or the pericardium invade the heart, interfere with its function, and produce heart failure. Such tumors can occasionally be diagnosed by special techniques but are seldom circumscribed enough to be removable by heart surgery. Occasionally intensive radiation treatment may temporarily control such tumors.

The most important form of heart tumor is *myxoma,* a loose, gelatine-like mass, usually developing in a cardiac atrium. There is still controversy as to whether it is a tumor or degenerated tissue, possibly from an old clot. Myxoma does not present itself as a malignant tumor and may remain without excessive growth for years. The important features of cardiac myxoma are two: (*a*) it may obstruct an orifice and imitate valvular stenosis (usually mitral); (*b*) small portions of the tumor may break loose and float with the stream of blood, producing emboli (such as strokes). Myxoma of the heart is usually curable by surgical treatment, and its proper recognition is of great practical importance.

MYXEDEMA HEART DISEASE

A specific form of heart disease occurs in several forms of thyroid gland deficiency (myxedema). As a result of the deficiency of thyroid hormone some metabolic or degenerative changes occur in the heart muscle which lead to cardiac enlargement and, sometimes, failure. In addition, fluid may accumulate in the pericardium and aggravate the cardiac difficulties. This type of heart disease usually develops when thyroid deficiency occurs spontaneously, but occasionally is produced by treatment of hyperthyroid states, either by operation or by destruction of the gland with radioactive iodine. Myxedema heart disease is curable by the administration of thyroid hormones.

"HYPERCIRCULATORY" STATES

It has been stated earlier that the heart responds with hypertrophy and later with failure to increased work load. Most of the conditions hitherto discussed dealt with increased work load due to elevated resistance (high pressure) or to increased flow through certain localized segments (valve incompetence, shunts). There are conditions, however, in which the *total* output of the heart has to be increased. Such states have been termed hypercirculatory states or high output states. Among such conditions, the two commonest are anemia and hyperthyroidism. In the former the number of red blood cells may be so low that tissues can be supplied with oxygen only if the total volume of blood reaching them increases. Thus increased cardiac output compensates for the low capacity for oxygen of the deficient blood. Cardiac output in severe anemia may be two or even three times the normal amount, which overloads the heart and may produce heart failure.

In hyperthyroidism the excess of thyroid hormone increases the metabolism of all cells of the body and thereby increases the demand for oxygen. These high demands lead to increase in cardiac output with effects upon the circulation similar to those of anemia. Both anemia and hyperthyroidism are usually correctable; their elimination reduces the cardiac work load and reestablishes normal cardiac function.

Other high output states include early stages of vitamin B deficiency states (beriberi heart disease), connections between an artery and a vein (arteriovenous fistula), and rare cases in which high cardiac output is present without a known cause.

CHRONIC PERICARDIAL DISEASE

The function of the pericardium is to facilitate the action of the heart by providing a "lubricant," pericardial fluid. Furthermore, it has a favorable action in restricting and confining the heart within its cavity, thereby preventing too sudden dilatation of it. The effect of the accumulation of excess fluid in the pericardial sac has already been discussed. Such an occurrence affects the heart acutely, for the pericardial sac is distensible and may gradually increase in size, as it does in the development of cardiac enlargement. However, when the pericardium becomes unduly thickened its responses may be different. The accumulation of fluid may be associated with continuous and prolonged interference with cardiac function; furthermore, the pericardium itself may become so thick that, like a coat of armor, it permanently envelops the heart in a rigid container and seriously impairs its work. Such a situation is called *constrictive pericarditis,* as opposed to *adhesive pericarditis,* where localized adhesions between the two layers of the pericardium develop. The latter form of pericardial disease is of no consequence to the circulation.

Constrictive pericarditis is usually a consequence of an active process, often in the distant past. The common forms of acute pericarditis, rheumatic and "benign," very seldom, if ever, produce constriction of the pericardial sac. The two common causes of pericardial constriction are: tuberculosis of the pericardium and inflammatory disease of the anterior portion of the thorax (mediastinum) involving the pericardium, caused by germs or injury. Occasionally constrictive pericarditis occurs without any clues as to its origin.

The essential effect of pericardial constriction upon the circulation is its interference with relaxation of the heart (diastole). Consequently, (*a*) the heart cannot fill properly, so that cardiac output is abnormally low, and (*b*) abnormally high pressure builds up in the atrium and the ventricle during diastole. Since low cardiac output and high atrial pressure are essential features of heart failure, constrictive pericarditis imitates and often masquerades as heart failure. The right ventricle is more often and more typically affected by the restrictive effects of pericardial constriction, so that signs of pericarditis include distention of veins in the neck, enlargement of the liver, accumulation of fluid in the abdominal cavity, and edema of the lower extremities—all signs of right ventricular failure. Signs of left ventricular failure—shortness of breath and congestion of the lungs—are uncommon.

The diagnosis of constrictive pericarditis can sometimes be made with great ease, particularly when calcium is deposited in the constricted pericardium and can be identified in the X-ray film. In some cases, however, the differential diagnosis between right-sided heart failure and constrictive pericarditis may be quite difficult and may not even be resolved by such complex diagnostic studies as cardiac catheterization or angiocardiography In rare cases exploratory operations have been performed without settling the diagnosis preoperatively.

Treatment of constrictive pericarditis is surgical. Although the surgeon can usually peel off the part of the thickened pericardium interfering to the greatest extent with cardiac function, complete cures cannot always be obtained, and improvement rather than cure is the usual result.

15

The Pulmonary Circulation and Its Abnormalities

The lungs represent a combination of a fuel filling station and exhaust deposit area for the circulation of blood. The importance of this organ is best emphasized by reminding the reader that the right side of the heart does nothing else but pump blood into and out of the lungs; since both sides of the heart pump the same amount of blood, the lungs receive as much blood as the entire remainder of the human body. The potential seriousness of disturbances of the pulmonary circulation is self-evident, but, as for other important organs (for example, the heart itself) nature has provided protective devices which minimize such disturbances. The most important disturbance of the circulation to the lungs is elevation of blood pressure within the lesser circulation (pulmonary hypertension). This disorder shows only a slight similarity to systemic hypertension (high blood pressure, chap. 11): rather than being caused by a faulty pressure regulatory mechanism, pulmonary hypertension can be caused by clots in the lungs, by excessive amounts of blood ejected into them, by "damming" of the blood at the other end of the pulmonary circulation, or by constriction of small blood vessels in the lungs. The mechanism causing such elevation of blood pressure in the lungs is of great importance, since some forms of pulmonary hypertension can be reversed and others cannot.

It has been emphasized in preceding chapters that the lesser circulation—pulmonary circulation—differs in many respects from the systemic circulation. To summarize these differences, it may be restated that the volume of blood ejected into the lungs—a single organ—equals that ejected into the aorta for the entire remainder of the body! Furthermore, pressure in the pulmonary circulation is influenced by many factors, in contrast to the systemic circulation, which is controlled solely by constriction and relaxation of the arterioles. Finally, the arterial pressure in the pulmonary circulation is roughly one-fifth that in the systemic circulation. With these differences it is not surprising that abnormalities affecting the pulmonary circulation are unlike those affecting other regions of the circulation.

Like that of its left-sided counterpart, the principal significance of disturbances of the pulmonary circulation is the imposition of an increased work load upon the right ventricle of the heart, which may produce its hypertrophy and failure. Such overload within this circuit is caused primarily by two mechanisms: increased blood flow to the lungs, and increased pressure within the pulmonary circulation. Increased blood flow is a characteristic feature of left-to-right shunts occurring almost exclusively in congenital heart disease. Their effects have been largely discussed in chapter 13. Pulmonary hypertension, also touched upon in previous chapters, involves the number one problem in disorders of the pulmonary circulation. This problem is of such magnitude and complexity that it will be presented here in its entirety at the risk of repeating some points already made.

PULMONARY HYPERTENSION

Our knowledge concerning pulmonary hypertension is relatively new: in contrast to the systemic arterial pressure, which can be measured by a simple apparatus, pressures within the pulmonary circulation can only be measured during cardiac catheterization. Consequently, a major procedure must be performed each time pressure in the pulmonary artery has to be obtained. Elevation of pressure in the pulmonary artery can be caused by one of three principal mechanisms: (1) increased resistance within the pulmonary vascular tree; (2) increased blood flow through the lungs; (3) increased pressure in the left atrium transmitted back through the pulmonary veins into the pulmonary arterial system. The main factors affecting these three mechanisms are:

1) Pulmonary hypertension owing to increased resistance within the pulmonary circulation may be caused by several factors. Spasm and constriction of the pulmonary arterioles—the only mechanism within the pulmonary circulation which is analogous to systemic hypertension—occurs in a variety of diseases. *Pulmonary arteriolar spasm* presents an important problem in treatment, and great efforts are being made to reveal circumstances under which spasm may be successfully eliminated, restoring more normal pressure in the pulmonary circulation. Other factors causing increased resistance include organic changes within the arterial tree, closing off some channels; occlusion of smaller branches of the pulmonary artery by emboli; and the sudden blockage of the main pulmonary artery or its principal branches by a large thrombus.

Pulmonary arteriolar spasm leading to pulmonary hypertension may be caused by specific stimuli. Two such stimuli have been discovered; their role in causing pulmonary hypertension is a considerable one. Such stimuli are: (*a*) reduced oxygen content in the blood (anoxia), such as occurs in high altitude, and (*b*) increased pressure within the left atrium characteristic of mitral stenosis and left ventricular failure. It has been demonstrated that pulmonary arteriolar spasm caused by these stimuli is reversible, so that their elimination will produce a fall in pulmonary artery pressure.

2) Pulmonary hypertension caused by increased blood flow to the lungs occurs almost entirely in congenital heart disease. An increase in blood flow within the pulmonary circulation does not automatically raise pressure within this circuit. The lungs have a large vascular reserve capacity which can accommodate excess blood without increasing resistance to flow. This occurs in normal individuals during exercise when cardiac output in-

creases (see chap. 3) without raising pressure in the pulmonary circulation. It has also been pointed out in chapter 13 that large shunts due to the various congenital communications between the two sides of the circulation may persist without elevation of pressure in the pulmonary circuit. However, for various reasons the reserve capacity of the pulmonary vascular tree may not be available in some cases of congenital heart disease, so that pulmonary arterial pressure rises in direct proportion to increases of pulmonary blood flow. This type of pulmonary hypertension occurring in congenital heart disease is called *hyperkinetic pulmonary hypertension*. Many of its ramifications have already been discussed.

3) Pressure transmitted backwards from the left atrium is termed *passive pulmonary hypertension*. High left atrial pressure occurring in mitral stenosis and in left ventricular failure dams up the blood flow and forces the right ventricle to eject blood under high pressure. This passive pulmonary hypertension is not to be confused with pulmonary arteriolar spasm (see above), which is also related to pressure rises in the left atrium and which occurs in some cases over and above the passive elevation of pressure.

Pulmonary hypertension presents problems to the physician different from those related to systemic arterial hypertension. The latter causes overloading of the left ventricle with its usual consequences, but it also may have such secondary serious effects as enhancement of atherosclerotic diseases of the coronary circulation and other regions, and damage to the kidney and brain. Such secondary effects do not exist in pulmonary hypertension, and its problems relate primarily to its effect upon the right ventricle. However, the challenge of pulmonary hypertension is that it occurs frequently in children and young individuals and produces serious disability earlier than systemic hypertension. The crucial question related to pulmonary hypertension is its reversibility. It has already been mentioned that some forms of it respond well to the elimination of its causative factor. Two forms of pulmonary hypertension would automatically be eliminated in such a manner: that related to excess flow, and that transmitted passively from the left atrium. Surgical closure of a left-to-right shunt associated with hyperkinetic pulmonary hypertension brings about an immediate fall in pulmonary artery pressure which can be measured on the operating room table. Similarly, relief of mitral stenosis producing fall in left atrial pressure immediately lowers pulmonary pressures. Other forms of reversible pulmonary hypertension are less dramatic and may require more time for a fall in pressures. These include pulmonary arteriolar spasm related to high left atrial pressure and to anoxia. Gradual fall in pulmonary arteriolar resistance occurs in some conditions after the elimination of these factors. Perhaps the most striking point about pulmonary hypertension is the fact that certain reversible forms of it may undergo transition into permanent forms. This occurs most frequently in congenital heart disease associated with high pulmonary blood flow, and is related to the development of organic diseases of the small pulmonary blood vessels. The importance of this self-perpetuating form of pulmonary hypertension has been discussed in connection with ventricular septal defect and other forms of congenital disease (chap. 13). Acknowledging that in congenital heart disease pulmonary hypertension is the most devastating factor reducing the life-span of children and young adults, the physician has to be acutely aware that a child may at one point have a reversible form of pulmonary hypertension and be a candidate for complete surgical cure, but a year or two later, if surgical treatment is postponed, may develop an inoperable form because of pulmonary vascular disease.

DISEASES AFFECTING THE
PULMONARY CIRCULATION

PULMONARY EMBOLISM

This is perhaps the most serious and unpredictable condition affecting the pulmonary circulation. It consists of occlusion of sections of the pulmonary arterial tree by thrombi wandering with the bloodstream from the venous part of the circulation or from the right side of the heart. The sites of formation of thrombi vary. While inflammatory diseases of the vein are usually associated with thrombosis (thrombophlebitis), pulmonary embolism occurs much more frequently in veins not affected by inflammation (phlebothrombosis). It is known that in susceptible individuals thrombi can form in veins, particularly during periods of inactivity. The veins most frequently affected by "silent" thrombosis are deep veins of the legs (*not* varicose veins) and veins in the pelvic organs (reproductive organs in women and prostatic veins in men). Because inactivity is an important cause of such thrombi, venous thrombosis and pulmonary emboli are particularly likely to occur in people who are bedridden.

There are four forms in which pulmonary embolism may occur:

1) Small single embolus affecting a segment of the lung which becomes clogged with blood—a condition termed *pulmonary infarct*. This is a relatively benign condition which may cause chest pain, spitting up blood, and some fever; it is shown on the chest X ray as a shadow similar to pneumonia; however, prompt recovery usually occurs in a single infarct without sequelae. The significance of pulmonary infarct lies in its implication that other, larger, and more serious emboli may develop from the source of the small embolus.

2) Large pulmonary embolism, or multiple emboli leading to overloading of the pulmonary circulation. When a certain area of the pulmonary arterial tree (usually more than half) is occluded by clots, pressure in the pulmonary artery rises. The sudden onset of pulmonary hypertension often does not permit time for adaptation and leads rapidly to right ventricular failure. Such an event, occasionally referred to as *acute cor pulmonale*, may be fatal, but it may reverse itself when pulmonary emboli are no longer forthcoming, either by cessation of thrombosis or in response to surgical intervention. Patients with acute cor pulmonale are very ill, and short of breath, may be in shock, and show the signs of right ventricular failure.

3) Massive pulmonary embolism causes death, usually instantly, without warning. It is the prevention of this dreaded complication which has placed so much emphasis upon signs of any disturbance of the venous circulation.

4) Small repeated pulmonary emboli may be feeding the pulmonary circulation over a period of weeks, months, or years, causing gradual elevation of pressure in the pulmonary artery and leading to chronic, irreversible pulmonary hypertension. Neither the course nor the points of origin of such emboli are known, but this mechanism is one of the important, though fortunately uncommon, forms of severe, usually fatal, pulmonary hypertension.

Treatment of pulmonary embolism depends upon circumstances. The physician has at his disposal anticoagulant therapy, which is quite effective in the prevention of further emboli (though it does not influence those already in the lungs); he can consider surgical treatment consisting of ligation (tying off) of veins suspected of feeding emboli (a large vein in the leg, or even the inferior vena cava); he can, finally, perform the heroic operation of removing a massive clot from the main pulmonary artery.

COR PULMONALE

This term literally means heart disease related to the lungs or pulmonary circulation; it should logically include all disturbances of the pulmonary circulation. However, in current medical terminology the term *chronic cor pulmonale* is used exclusively to indicate the cardiac effect of chronic diseases of the lungs. Acute cor pulmonale has already been mentioned as referring to large pulmonary embolism, but there are some who question the use of the term "cor pulmonale" in connection with anything but diseases of the lungs.

Not all diseases of the lungs affect the heart. Acute diseases, such as pneumonia, have no consistent effect upon the heart. Tuberculosis seldom produces untoward effects upon the heart or the pulmonary circulation. Three diseases of the lungs have important bearing upon the pulmonary circulation: pulmonary emphysema, chronic pulmonary fibrosis, and severe deformities of the thorax. The principal effect of these conditions upon the heart is pulmonary hypertension. The main cause of pulmonary hypertension is anoxia, low oxygen tension in the arterial blood. An additional factor is thought to be the destruction of lung tissue by some of these diseases, which might eliminate enough pulmonary blood vessels to create higher resistance to blood flow.

Emphysema is by far the commonest cause of chronic cor pulmonale. Interference with oxygenation of blood in the lungs occurs usually in advanced stages of emphysema, when pulmonary hypertension makes itself evident, leading eventually to right ventricular failure. Most patients with emphysema die of heart failure. It has been mentioned that pulmonary hypertension due to anoxia is caused by spasm of arterioles and is reversible. In some stages of emphysema improved lung function may abolish anoxia and temporarily reverse pulmonary hypertension. However, the course of emphysema is such that eventually anoxia is continuously present and pulmonary hypertension becomes irreversible. The other diseases of the lungs and thorax affect the pulmonary circulation in a similar manner.

There are a few reversible causes of chronic cor pulmonale, but they are quite rare. Among these is chronic mountain sickness, an exaggerated response of some individuals' pulmonary vasculature to high altitude, which may be reversed by moving the patient to sea level. Another condition is represented by decreased ventilation of lungs due to extreme obesity, which may cause anoxia and pulmonary hypertension and which can be reversed by loss of body weight. As a rule, however, chronic cor pulmonale is a serious disease representing late stages of lung disease. Treatment is limited to controlling heart failure and is usually not very effective. The duration of illness from the time right heart failure is evident is relatively short, with death occurring within a few months or a very few years.

PRIMARY PULMONARY HYPERTENSION

This is a rare disease, usually affecting young individuals and occasionally children, in which severe, progressive pulmonary hypertension develops without a known cause. Its onset is inconspicuous, with slowly developing limitation of activities from excessive tiredness and shortness of breath. Signs of pulmonary hypertension can be recognized by examination, X ray, and electrocardiography. Cardiac catheterization has to be performed to rule out the possibility of secondary pulmonary hypertension (see below). Patients may live for several years partly incapacitated, but sooner or later heart failure supervenes.

The difficulty of separating primary pulmonary hypertension from cases of pulmonary hypertension due to small pulmonary emboli has already been mentioned. The similarity between the two conditions is considerable, and often they cannot be told apart until after death.

OTHER DISEASES ASSOCIATED WITH PULMONARY HYPERTENSION

The three conditions discussed above cause pulmonary hypertension, which is their primary link with heart disease. There are a number of diseases of the heart in which pulmonary hypertension develops secondarily, and is only one of several factors affecting the heart. These conditions have already been discussed and will merely be mentioned here. They are: (*a*) many forms of congenital heart disease, (*b*) mitral stenosis and mitral insufficiency, and (*c*) chronic failure of the left ventricle of the heart.

These conditions may produce all three types of pulmonary hypertension: passive, hyperkinetic, and that related to high pulmonary vascular resistance. However, the first two types are less likely to cause severe pulmonary hypertension than the third. Consequently, in ordinary clinical terms the concept of "pulmonary hypertension" is most often applied to elevated pulmonary vascular resistance. Thus, pulmonary hypertension in connection with mitral stenosis connotes that, in addition to passive elevation of pressure in the pulmonary artery, arteriolar constriction has taken place. In congenital heart disease, separating operable cases with high flow (hyperkinetic) from inoperable cases with high resistance constitutes the basic problem (see chap. 13).

16

Diseases of the Blood Vessels

The heart is the central organ of the circulatory system, and its function is intimately related to other components of this system. The reader is already aware of the fact that two of the most important disturbances of the heart in reality are diseases of the blood vessels: coronary disease and hypertension. In this chapter a brief discussion of diseases of the major blood vessels is presented, with special reference to those customarily included in the general term "cardiovascular diseases."

ATHEROSCLEROTIC DISEASE OF THE ARTERIES

The subject of atherosclerosis was discussed in detail in chapter 10 with reference to its causes and mechanisms and its relation to coronary artery disease. In practical terms atherosclerosis is universally equated with coronary artery disease, for it represents the most serious, the most spectacular, and the commonest manifestation of atherosclerosis as a cause of human disease. However, occlusive atherosclerotic disease of other arteries also plays an important, even if lesser, role.

As in coronary diseases, atherosclerotic occlusive disease of other arteries is a gradual process, which occasionally may be accelerated by formation of a thrombus. The difference between coronary atherosclerosis and that afflicting peripheral blood vessels, however, is that thrombi occluding the coronary artery

267

almost always originate within the affected artery; those occluding peripheral arteries frequently arise from emboli. Gradual occlusion of any blood vessel produces important adjusting mechanisms in the form of "detours." These may already be available, for in some regions of the circulation alternate channels are normally present. The best-known example of this mechanism is the radial artery, the customary site of palpating the pulse at the wrist, which can be occluded, or tied off, without any untoward consequences, for blood can reach the entire hand through the ulnar artery (running on the other side of the wrist). Thus, the consequences of atherosclerotic occlusive disease of the arteries depends on how well a given region can be supplied with blood through alternate passages. The most important regions, next to the coronary circulation, in which atherosclerotic disease causes major problems are three: the brain, the kidneys, and the lower extremities.

ATHEROSCLEROTIC DISEASES OF THE BRAIN

Some of the most serious forms of damage to the brain, including various forms of "strokes," are caused by circulatory disturbances in the brain. These fall into three categories: hemorrhage in the brain due to rupture of a major blood vessel; occlusion of an artery by atherosclerotic changes; and occlusion of an artery by an embolus arriving with the bloodstream from a distance.

In recent years there has been a change in emphasis in relation to atherosclerotic occlusive diseases of the brain, which was due, in part, to improvement of surgical methods for treatment of cerebral arterial disease, and in part to refinement of contrast visualization of cerebral circulation. It became apparent that a significant number of cases of cerebral vascular disease are not due to atherosclerosis within the brain substance itself, but to total or even partial occlusion of the arteries in the neck leading to the brain. Consequently, in suitable cases, selective angiograms are being performed which can outline the condition of the four principal arteries supplying the brain. The feasibility of surgical treatment depends entirely on whether the occlusive disease is located in an accessible or an inaccessible portion of these arteries.

Surgical treatment consisting of removal or bypassing of blocks in accessible arteries is the only hopeful approach to the problem of strokes and other forms of cerebral damage ("treatment" usually means prevention of further damage, for improvement of cerebral circulation will not affect the damage already done). Medical methods using various drugs and anticoagulant therapy have not been definitely proven to be of benefit.

ATHEROSCLEROTIC DISEASE OF THE KIDNEYS

Occlusive disease of the renal circulation and its relationship to "essential" hypertension has been discussed in chapter 11.

ATHEROSCLEROTIC DISEASE OF LOWER EXTREMITIES

Disturbances of the circulation to the lower extremities are very common, but only in a relatively small number of patients are significant consequences detectable. The effects vary from minor disturbance to total interruption of the circulation, leading to gangrene. The principal symptom is pain. In the early stages pain occurs with exercise, similar to anginal pain in coronary artery disease. During increased demands upon the muscles when walking, narrowed arteries are incapable of supplying enough blood and the individual experiences pain in the exercising muscles which necessitates interruption of exercise. This type of pain is called *intermittent claudication* (recurrent limping due to pain in the legs). In more severe disturbances of the circulation, pain in the extremity may occur at rest as well. Another consequence of impaired circulation is increased proneness to infection from minor cuts and injuries. Furthermore, large ulcers (*ischemic leg ulcers*) may appear on the extremities; they are exceedingly difficult to heal. Gangrene signifies complete absence of nutrition to a certain area; it is rather uncommon in progressive atherosclerotic occlusive diseases, and is more often encountered in the sudden total occlusion due to embolism.

Occlusive disease of the lower extremities is primarily a disease of old age, but may occur in middle age as well. It is particularly common in individuals with diabetes; high proneness to peripheral vascular disease, with secondary infections and possibility of gangrene, are well known in this disease. Good control of diabetes may somewhat reduce the probability of such complications, but by no means prevents its occurrence altogether. There are forms of occlusive vascular disease of the lower extremities which suggest an inflammatory nature of the process and which may involve the veins as well as the arteries. Such forms, occurring in younger individuals, have been called *thromboangiitis obliterans* (Buerger's disease). There is currently a controversy as to whether such cases should be separated from atherosclerosis as another disease, or merely considered its variant.

Treatment of atherosclerosis of the lower extremities has undergone considerable changes in recent years, largely because of better diagnostic and surgical techniques. At present selective angiography can show details of the architecture of vascular changes in the lower extremities. In an unexpectedly large number of cases the major occlusive process has been found in a surgically accessible area, such as the lower part of the aorta and its larger branches, interjecting a note of hope by permitting surgical relief.

The success of the treatment of occlusive disease of lower extremities varies considerably. Medical methods are generally ineffective; many drugs purported to have the effect of dilating blood vessels have been used, but few have been definitely proven to be effective. Surgical interruption of the lower part of the sympathetic nervous chain (lumbar sympathectomy) has been used widely with equivocal results. This method is now less popular because of more effective direct methods of attack. Surgical treatment of occlusive disease involves two methods of approach: removal of the occluding part from the inside of the vessel (*endarterectomy*), and replacement of portions of the artery with synthetic grafts. This method is primarily suited to cases with occlusion in the lower abdominal aorta and its large branches. The effectiveness of such surgery is variable. Spectacular successes are sometimes achieved but disappointing results are not infrequent, because of reocclusion of the arteries and spread of the disease to arteries below the operated area.

OTHER FORMS OF ATHEROSCLEROSIS

Occlusive disease of the upper extremities is very rare. Insignificant degrees of it may account for differences in blood pressure when taken in the arms. Significant disturbances of the circulation are almost always related to complete occlusion from embolism. Rarely, occlusive disease may affect the abdominal organs and cause intermittent pain (*angina abdominalis*). More serious disturbances, here too, are almost always related to embolism. The effects of atherosclerotic disease upon the aorta will be discussed in the section on aneurysm.

THROMBOEMBOLIC DISEASE

Thromboembolism has been discussed throughout previous chapters but will be briefly recapitulated here. The essence of this process is the formation of thrombi within the cardiovascular system, which then are torn loose from the wall upon which they form and travel with the bloodstream until they reach a blood vessel of the proper size, which they fill completely. The pathway of these thrombi varies; some lodge in the brain, others in the leg, and so on. Thromboembolism occurs in both sides of the circulation, venous and arterial.

Embolic disease in the arterial system has three main sources: (*a*) thrombi forming upon the wall of the left atrium in atrial fibrillation; (*b*) thrombi forming on the wall of the left ventricle, usually caused by a recent myocardial infarction; and (*c*) thrombi originating from heart valves in bacterial endocarditis. Rarely, thrombi may tear loose from atherosclerotic plaques in the aorta and cause emboli.

An embolus lodged in an artery abruptly stops the circulation of blood. As stated, the effect of this depends on how well the given organ or part of the body is supplied by alternate channels. In areas where adequate collateral channels are not available, an embolus may have serious consequences. An embolus within an organ (brain, heart, kidney, lung, spleen) usually produces an *infarct* (death of tissue deprived of blood supply). Embolism within a larger artery (aorta, artery to extremities) may produce signs of disturbed circulation to a whole region. Embolic occlusion occurs with dramatic suddenness. Severe pain in the affected area occurs in occlusion in the abdomen or extremities. Cerebral embolism often causes sudden loss of consciousness with or without associated stroke. Patients may go into shock. If embolism occludes an artery to an extremity, the affected extremity, in addition to being painful, becomes pale and cold.

The diagnosis of embolism is usually obvious, particularly when the underlying condition is an acute one (endocarditis, myocardial infarction). Special diagnostic techniques are rarely necessary. The most important decision the physician has to make applies to those forms of embolism for which surgical treatment is necessary. Obviously, embolic strokes are not suited to any direct attack. Occlusion of the arterial circulation to an extremity poses a real problem, for surgical removal of such an embolus may save that extremity from gangrene. However, such surgical attack is not always necessary, since partial restoration of the circulation may develop via the collateral channels within hours and may eventually become adequate as a permanent source of blood supply. Patients with arterial embolism thus have to be watched very carefully; the decision of the point at which to undertake surgical removal of the embolus is a difficult one and requires mature judgment on the part of the physician.

Nonemergency treatment of arterial embolism includes rest and proper conditions enhancing healing, and is primarily directed toward preventing future emboli. Anticoagulant treatment of myocardial infarction and of atrial fibrillation for the prevention of emboli has already been discussed. Such therapy is not suitable for bacterial endocarditis, though. Here prompt and vigorous treatment of the infection may prevent embolization.

Thromboembolism on the venous side of the circulation leading to pulmonary infarcts and other sequelae has been discussed in chapter 15. In congenital heart disease and in other conditions in which there are communications between the two sides of the heart, thrombi from the venous side of the circulation may occasionally bypass the lung and produce embolism in the arterial circulation. This is termed *paradoxical embolism.*

ANEURYSMS OF THE AORTA

Aneurysm of the aorta is a localized bulge, an outpouching of a wall of the aorta due to weakness of its wall. While it affects smaller arteries as well, the aorta is the principal site of this serious form of arterial disease. A special form of aneurysm, *dissecting aneurysm,* will be discussed separately. There are three principal causes of aortic aneurysm: (*a*) syphilis, (*b*) atherosclerosis, and (*c*) trauma (injury). Syphilitic aneurysm almost always affects the ascending aorta or the aortic arch. In the past this was the commonest form of aortic aneurysm, but the reduction in the incidence of syphilis, and the effective methods of treatment preventing its late consequences (among which is aneurysm), have made this form of aneurysm a rarity. Atherosclerosis is now by far the leading cause of aneurysms. Atherosclerotic aneurysms are commoner in the abdominal aorta than in the thoracic aorta.

The size of the aneurysm varies from a gentle, blisterlike outpouching of a wall of the aorta to huge tumors filling most of the abdominal cavity. Aneurysms, as a rule, do not affect the circulation in any way, so that uninterrupted flow of blood occurs through the structure. They produce no symptoms except, rarely, that when reaching large size they may press on some body structures and produce pain. The diagnosis of aneurysm is made, as a rule, by finding it during routine examination: X-ray examination of the chest will reveal the presence of aneurysm in the thorax, while physical examination of the abdomen will demonstrate abdominal aneurysms which present themselves as pulsating masses.

It has been stated that an aneurysm usually produces no signs or symptoms and that most individuals are unaware of its existence. Its principal significance lies in the possibility of rupture of an aneurysm. Rupture of a thoracic aneurysm almost always causes instantaneous death. Abdominal aneurysm may rupture more gradually, seeping blood but allowing, on occasion, enough time to perform an emergency operation.

Treatment of aortic aneurysm is limited to surgical resection (or cutting off) of the outpouching. Great progress has been made in recent years in this field, and the risk of such surgery is comparatively small. Thoracic aneurysms are more difficult to resect, particularly if they involve the ascending aorta. However, now, with the aid of artificial circulation through a pump-oxygenator, even this type of aneurysm can be excised. Abdominal aneurysms require relatively simpler methods. Almost all aneurysms require replacement of the arterial wall by artificial grafts.

Aneurysm due to injuries (such as automobile accidents) presents a somewhat better outlook for surgical correction, since the aorta is usually in good condition, as opposed to atherosclerotic aneurysms where the vessel above or below the bulging area may be damaged as well.

The principal problem in treatment of aortic aneurysms is the selection of cases for surgery. The process of selection has to be based upon guessing the chances of rupture of an aneurysm (depending on its size and location) as against the risk of the operation. Even now, with improvement in technique, such a decision may be very difficult, particularly when aneurysms develop in patients in their 70's and 80's, who are particularly prone to this disease.

Dissecting aneurysm is a special type of aneurysm which bears little relationship to ordinary aneurysms. In dissecting aneurysms there is an inherent weakness in the middle layer of the aorta, which tends to separate the outer and the inner layer from each other. A dissecting aneurysm is formed when the intima (inner layer) of the aorta tears and blood finds a way between the inner layers and the remainder of the aorta. In such cases blood has two channels: some of it flows normally within the intima, the "inner tube," and some between two of the three layers of the aorta. Somewhere, there is another tear in the intima through which the blood returns. Usually the initial tear is above the aortic valves, and the lower tear in the abdominal aorta. This "double-channel aorta" has two possible effects upon the circulation: the dissection may progress down to the aortic valve and produce aortic valve insufficiency by distorting the aortic orifice, or the dissection may occlude the exits of some tributaries from the aorta and produce vascular occlusion (similar to embolism). The main danger, however, is from rupture of a vessel, since blood flow under the normally high pressure is separated from the outside by only one or two layers of tissue instead of three.

Dissecting aneurysm occurs suddenly; it may or may not be brought on by an injury which is often trivial in itself. The cause of it lies in a deficient structure of the media (intermediate layer) of the aorta. This layer, in certain individuals, becomes dead (necrotic), hence the term *medionecrosis aortica cystica*. Such abnormality of the structure of the aorta may be hereditary, associated with other structural abnormalities of connective tissue in the body (Marfan's syndrome). Occasionally major trauma, such as a severe blow to the chest, may dissect the layers in a normal aorta.

Dissecting aneurysm is a serious disease and may lead to death either instantly or within a matter of hours, before arrangement for the rather involved surgical treatment can be made. A fair proportion of cases, however, survive the initial attack (which is occasionally mistaken for a "coronary"), after which surgical treatment can be undertaken. Such treatment has been increasingly successful in recent years, particularly with the use of circulatory bypass (partial or complete, with an artificial heart–lung machine).

DISEASES OF VEINS

VARICOSE VEINS

Varicose veins are the commonest disease of veins and one of the commonest human disorders. Their cause is not entirely understood; it is thought that they may be related to some inherent weakness of the vein wall. Their formation is facilitated by gravity, which subjects the column of blood in the legs to a pressure of 75 to 100 mm. Hg. The common variety of varicose veins involves the irregular enlargement of superficial veins running alongside the inner surface of the leg. Varicose veins may also involve the deep veins of the leg and intermediate veins, providing abnormal communication between the superficial and deep veins. The effect of varicose veins upon the circulation is relatively minor. Even though blood flows very slowly in these wormlike venous structures and formation of thrombi is quite common, blood returning from the legs can take alternate channels. Emboli originating from clots in varicose veins are very rare. Occasionally, extensive varicose veins may interfere sufficiently with return of blood from the legs to cause edema of the ankles. Very occasionally, impaired nutrition of the skin in the affected areas may lead to the formation of superficial skin ulcers. Varicose veins are aggravated by any factor obstructing the return of blood from the legs: the pregnant uterus is a common factor precipitating varicose veins. Also, workers required to stand motionless for long periods of time (cooks, barbers) are more prone to varicose veins than are other individuals.

Treatment of varicose veins is not always necessary. In many cases treatment is requested for cosmetic rather than medical reasons. Treatment of small, superficial veins may consist of injecting the varicosities with a chemical substance which makes them shrink and disappear. Elastic bandages and stockings help the circulation in cases where surgical treatment is not undertaken. More extensive varicosities require surgical treatment, or ligation (tying off the vessels).

In addition to affecting veins of the legs, varicosities may form in other parts of the body to compensate for occlusive disease in the venous circulation. They are a venous equivalent of the "collateral channels" of the arterial circulation. The best-known secondary varicose veins occur in cirrhosis of the liver (affecting the veins of the abdominal wall, the esophagus, and the rectum); in occlusive disease of the inferior vena cava (large varicosities along the sides of the abdominal wall); and occlusive disease of the superior vena cava (varicosities of veins in the arm and upper superficial veins of the chest).

THROMBOPHLEBITIS AND PHLEBOTHROMBOSIS

These processes have been mentioned in connection with pulmonary embolism. Thrombophlebitis is a painful swelling of the vein due to inflammatory disease, usually associated with inflammation of tissues around the veins. Thrombophlebitis of lesser veins may be a trivial illness requiring a few days in bed, but disease of deeper veins may be serious. Thrombophlebitis may occur without detectable cause, and may be a response to minor injuries. A particularly serious form of thrombophlebitis is inflammatory disease caused by bacterial infection (*septic thrombophlebitis*), which may be a manifestation of generalized sepsis. Thrombophlebitis may be the source of serious pulmonary emboli, but is decidedly less common than the noninflammatory phlebothrombosis. Treatment of thrombophlebitis consists of bed rest, anticoagulant therapy, and antibiotics, if they are indicated.

Phlebothrombosis, already discussed in chapter 15, is one of the most unpredictable and potentially serious disorders of the venous circulation, since it involves the formation of large thrombi, which are particularly prone to float along with the bloodstream and cause pulmonary emboli, often fatal. Phlebothrombosis may develop inconspicuously, without any warning symptoms. Treatment, as indicated, is anticoagulation or surgical ligation of the affected vein.

ARTERIOVENOUS FISTULA

This is a very interesting disease which affects the circulation in a local, circumscribed area but has consequences concerning the heart and the entire circulation. Arteriovenous fistula represents a connection (or a series of connections) between a major artery and vein. It may be congenital or acquired. Congenital arteriovenous fistula may occur in any part of the body, including the inside of the skull. It may be a simple communication between an artery and a vein or, more frequently, may take the form of a congenital vascular tumor (*hemangioma*), which consists of millions of small connections between arteries and veins and has the same effect upon the circulation as a single connection. Acquired arteriovenous fistula is almost always due to injury and is particularly likely to occur after stab and gunshot wounds.

An arteriovenous fistula of reasonable size will provide an outlet from the closed arterial system through which the blood will be drained into the low-pressure venous system. The effect of this is an increase in blood flow to compensate for the blood escaping into the fistula. Not unlike patent ductus arteriosus, the blood flow may have to be increased up to three times the normal value, for two-thirds of the blood returns to the vein without reaching the tissues. Thus, arteriovenous fistula overloads the entire circulation, as both ventricles participate in it. The heart often hypertrophies, dilates, and then fails unless the fistula is surgically closed.

The diagnosis of arteriovenous fistula can usually be made by a characteristic murmur produced at the site of the communication. The effects of the fistula upon the circulation can be surmised by the type of pulse and the size of the heart. Surgical closure can be performed in all accessible areas and usually presents no major problems for experienced vascular surgeons.

An interesting form of arteriovenous fistula is located in the lungs. This is almost always due to congenital hemangioma. In this form of fistula blood is shunted from the pulmonary artery to the pulmonary vein. Even though the low pressure in the pulmonary system does not lend itself to the same generalized consequences and overloading of the heart does not occur, the mixture of "blue" blood from the pulmonary artery directly entering the pulmonary vein and bypassing the lungs is equivalent to a right-to-left shunt and causes cyanosis which may be intense.

Glossary

Addison's disease.   A disease caused by destruction of the adrenal glands, characterized by weakness, low blood pressure, and brown pigmentation of the skin.

Aldosterone.   An adrenal gland hormone regulating salt and water balance of body tissues.

Alveolus.   The air cell of the lung.

Amyloidosis.   A disease in which an abnormal protein substance, amyloid, is deposited in various tissues. *Cardiac amyloidosis*, abnormal deposition of amyloid in the heart muscle.

Aneurysm.   An abnormal outpouching of a wall of the heart or a blood vessel (commonly affecting the aorta).

Angina pectoris.   A term for attacks of chest pain caused by inadequate blood supply to the heart muscle.

Angiocardiography.   A diagnostic procedure consisting of injection of a contrast substance into the vascular system in order to outline details of the heart and blood vessels in simultaneously taken X-ray films.

Angiography.   Same procedure as angiocardiography except taken for study of blood vessels only.

Anticoagulant.   A drug or agent hindering the clotting of blood, used primarily to prevent blood from clotting inside blood vessels.

Antistreptolysin titer.   A blood test in which antibodies against the streptococcus are measured; used to determine whether a

281

person had a streptococcal infection in the recent past.

Arrest, cardiac. Sudden stoppage of the circulation of blood due to cessation of effective heart action.

Arrhythmia. A disturbance of the regular sequence of heart-beats.

Arteriosclerosis. "Hardening of the arteries," a broad term connoting the over-all degenerative diseases of the arteries in the body.

Arteriole. A small branch of the arterial system, barely visible to the naked eye.

Arteriovenous. Connecting an artery and a vein. Arteriovenous fistula, an abnormal connection between a large artery and a large vein.

Artery. A thick-walled blood vessel transporting blood away from the heart under high pressure.

Ascites. Abnormal accumulation of serous fluid in the abdominal cavity.

Asthma. A form of shortness of breath, usually episodic, characterized by wheezing and related to spasms of the smaller bronchial tubes.

Ataxia. A disease of the brain causing lack of muscular coordination and particularly affecting the gait. *Friedreich's ataxia,* a disease of the central nervous system in which the heart may be involved.

Atherosclerosis. Disease of the medium-sized arteries in which there is a tendency to narrowing of the vessel's passages.

Atresia. Closure or absence of a normal body orifice. *Pulmonary atresia, tricuspid atresia,* congenital defects in which the pulmonary or tricuspid orifices of the heart are totally closed.

Atrioventricular. Connecting an atrium and a ventricle. *Atrioventricular block,* an abnormality of conduction in which the impulse from the atrium is delayed or incapable of reaching the ventricle. *Atrioventricular node,* a part of the conducting system of the heart located at the border between the atria and the ventricles. *Atrioventricular valve*, one of the two inflow valves of the ventricles of the heart.

Atrium. One of the two thin-walled upper chambers of the heart.

Auscultation. The act of listening to the sound of the heart, lungs, or other organs, usually with the aid of the stethoscope.

Autonomic. Self-regulating. *Autonomic nervous system*, a system of nerves throughout the body distributed to the heart and blood vessels and various other organs, which regulates involuntary functions of these structures.

Ballistocardiography. Graphic registration of motion of the body generated with each heartbeat.

Basal metabolism. The energy needed to maintain life functions in a resting, completely relaxed individual.

Beriberi. A disease, prevalent mostly in the tropics, consisting of metabolic disturbances due to deficiency in vitamin B_1 in the diet. Beriberi heart disease, heart disease caused by vitamin B_1 deficiency.

Bigeminal rhythm. A disturbance of heart rhythm in which two beats are close together and are followed by a longer pause, the second beat usually being ectopic, or displaced.

Bundle branch. One of two divisional branches of the bundle of His, the left one supplying the left ventricle, the right one the right ventricle.

Bundle-branch block. An abnormal condition of the conducting system interrupting .conduction through one of the two bundle branches.

Bundle of His. Part of the conducting system of the heart, transmitting the impulse from the atrioventricular node down to the ventricle.

Calcific. Containing deposits of calcium; in heart disease, often applied to obstructive disease of the valve, e.g. calcific aortic stenosis.

Capillary. Thinnest, hairlike components of the vascular system, visible only by microscopy.

Carditis.   Inflammatory disease of the heart involving all three layers of the heart, and usually a manifestation of rheumatic fever.

Catheterization.   Insertion of a thin tube ("catheter") through a passage into an organ of the body. *Cardiac catheterization*, insertion of the tube through a vein or an artery into the cavity of the heart.

Chorda tendinea (usually pl., *chordae tendineae*).   Cordlike structure fastened to the edges of the mitral and tricuspid valves of the heart, which facilitates valve action.

Chorea.   A disease of the central nervous system manifested by involuntary uncoordinated motion of parts of the body; the commonest form is that occuring in rheumatic fever and popularly referred to as "St. Vitus' dance."

Coarctation.   Narrowing of a major artery. *Coarctation of the aorta*, congenital malformation, usually of the arch of the aorta, consisting of a localized narrowing of that vessel.

Collateral circulation.   Blood supply reaching a certain organ or part of the body in a roundabout way rather than through normal channels, usually because of blockage of normal supply channels.

Compensation.   Term applied in connection with heart failure: a state in which an increased work load upon the heart can be managed without major disturbance of heart function.

Concentric.   Term applied to hypertrophy: increase in thickness of the heart muscle without increase in the total size of the heart; opposite to "excentric."

Conducting system.   A system of specialized cells on the inside of the heart which transmit impulses from one part of the heart to another. See also Atrioventricular node; Bundle branch; Bundle of His; Sinoatrial node.

Congestion.   Excessive accumulation of blood in an organ or a region of the body.

Conjunctiva.   Membrane lining the eyelids and the front part of the eyeball.

Coronary.   Pertaining to the blood supply of the heart itself.

Coronary artery, artery supplying the heart. *Coronary vein*, vein draining the heart. *Coronary occlusion*, complete closure of a major coronary artery, usually by clot (coronary thrombosis).

Cor pulmonale. Heart disease caused by certain disturbances of the pulmonary circulation.

Cushing's disease or syndrome. A disease caused by malfunction of the pituitary gland or adrenal gland and characterized by obesity and high blood pressure.

Cyanosis. Bluish color of the body, particularly lips and fingertips, due to lowered content of oxygen in the blood reaching the skin.

Decompensation. Term applied in connection with heart failure: a state in which an increased work load upon the heart can no longer be managed and heart failure results.

Depolarization. Discharge of electricity by heart muscle cells occurring just before contraction of the heart.

Diastasis. A stage of the heart cycle: part of the relaxation period (diastole) during which little blood flow occurs.

Diastole. A stage of the heart cycle: the entire period of relaxation of the heart muscle.

Dissecting aneurysm. A special form of aneurysm in which two coats of the aorta or another major artery separate and blood seeps between them.

Dissociation. A disturbance of conduction of the cardiac impulse during which the atria and ventricles beat independently of each other, not necessarily because of interruption of pathways connecting them.

Diuretic. A drug increasing the flow of urine, usually administered for the elimination of excess body fluids.

Ductus arteriosus. An arterial vessel connecting the aorta and the pulmonary artery in the fetus. This channel normally closes after birth. Its failure to close leads to a malformation, patent ductus arteriosus.

Dyspnea. The patient's awareness of being short of breath.

Dystrophy. Faulty nutrition. *Muscular dystrophy*, a group of diseases affecting the skeletal muscles in which the heart may be involved.

Ectopic. Displaced. *Ectopic rhythm*, origin of heartbeat from a region other than the normal pacemaker.

Edema. Abnormal accumulation of serous fluid in the loose tissues under the skin, causing puffy swelling of various parts of the body.

Effort dyspnea. Shortness of breath in response to performance of exercise.

Effusion. Accumulation of serous fluid in a body cavity, as pleural effusion, pericardial effusion.

Electrocardiogram. Record of electric potential generated during heart action.

Embolus. A plug of abnormal material (usually a clot) transferred with the flow of blood from one part of the circulation to another and lodged so as to obstruct blood flow within an artery.

Emphysema. A disease of the lungs associated with their hyperinflation and faulty ventilation and secondarily affecting the heart.

Encephalopathy. An abnormal condition of the brain. *Hypertensive encephalopathy*, disturbance of brain function occurring in severe hypertension.

Endarteritis. The inflammatory disease of the inner layer of an artery.

Endocardium. The inner coat lining the heart. Endocarditis, inflammatory disease of that layer.

Epicardium. The outer coat of the heart; one of the two parts of the pericardium.

Erythema. Skin rash consisting of uniform redness of the skin.

Essential hypertension. Hypertension of undetermined origin.

Etiology. The cause, origin, and factors contributing to the development of a disease or abnormal condition.

Excentric. Term applied to hypertrophy of the heart: increase in thickness of the heart muscle associated with increase in size of the cavity; opposite to "concentric."

Extracellular. Outside the cells. *Extracellular fluid*, tissue fluid outside the cells.

Extrasystole. A disturbance of the rhythm of the heart caused by a heartbeat occurring out of sequence.

Fibrillation. Uncoordinated twitching of heart muscle leading to loss of function of the affected chambers (atrial fibrillation, ventricular fibrillation).

Fibrosis. Replacement of the normal tissue of an organ or region of the body with fibrous tissue (scar tissue).

Fluoroscopy. Examination with the aid of the X-ray machine in which the image is inspected on a screen rather than photographed.

Flutter. Rapid, semicoordinated twitching of a heart chamber associated with partial loss of function (atrial flutter, ventricular flutter).

Foramen ovale. Opening between the two atria normally present in the fetus and closed after birth, but occasionally remains open (patent).

Fossa ovalis. An oval niche in the wall of the atrium representing the closed remnant of the foramen ovale.

Ganglion. A collection of nerve cells, particularly important in the function of the autonomic nervous system. *Ganglionic blocking agents*, a group of drugs blocking transmission of such nervous impulses across ganglions and thereby altering many involuntary functions of the body.

Glomerulonephritis. Inflammatory disease of the kidney, often associated with hypertension.

Glycogen storage disease. A metabolic abnormality causing the deposition of an excess of glycogen (starchlike carbohydrate, normally stored in moderate quantities in the liver and other organs as reserve fuel) in various organs including the heart, where it alters the function of such organs.

Gradient. A difference in pressure between two points of the circulation.

Hemolysis. The process of breakdown of the wall of the red blood cell causing the cell contents to spill into blood plasma.

Humoral. Pertaining to "humors" of the body: chemical agents mediating certain regulatory functions, as opposed to "nervous" or "neurogenic" regulation.

Hypercirculatory. Associated with increased volume of the circulation.

Hyperkinetic. Associated with increased motion. *Hyperkinetic pulmonary hypertension,* pulmonary hypertension caused by excessive blood flow to the lungs.

Hypertension. Elevated pressure, usually referring to high arterial blood pressure.

Hypertrophy. Excessive growth of a muscle or organ; when applied to the heart, increased mass of heart muscle, usually related to increased work load.

Idiopathic. Of undetermined cause.

Infarction. An area of damage to an organ resulting from stoppage of blood flow to that area.

Infundibulum. Funnel-like structure. Infundibulum of the right ventricle, the outflow portion of that ventricle leading to the pulmonary artery.

Insufficiency, valvular. Faulty function of a heart valve permitting backflow of blood.

Intima. Inner layer of a blood vessel.

Ischemia. Local deficiency in blood supply due to obstruction or spasm of the supplying artery. *Myocardial ischemia,* reduced blood supply to a portion of the heart muscle leading to significant symptoms of heart disease.

Isometric. Pertaining to change in tension of a muscle without change in size, for example, isometric contraction and relaxation of the heart muscle.

Leukocytosis. Increased number of white blood cells.

Media. Middle layer of a blood vessel.

Mediosclerosis. Degenerative disease selectively involving the middle layer of the arteries.

Membranous septum. Part of the partition between the ventricles of the heart in which a thin membrane rather than muscle separates the two chambers.

Minute volume. The amount of blood ejected by a ventricle of the heart in one minute.

Mitral. Pertaining to the valve separating the left atrium and the left ventricle ("mitral valve").

Mural thrombus. A clot adhering to a wall of the heart or large artery (not carried from a distance).

Myocardiopathy. Disease of the heart muscle, regardless of whether inflammatory or not. Also called *cardiomyopathy.*

Myocarditis. Inflammatory disease of the heart muscle.

Myocardium. Muscular layer of the heart; heart muscle.

Myxedema. Disease caused by a serious deficiency in thyroid gland hormone.

Myxoma. Benign tumor of the heart formed of a gelatin-like substance.

Necrosis. Death of living tissue. Myocardial necrosis, death of heart muscle due to local inadequacy of blood supply.

Neurogenic. Regulated by nervous impulses; term used primarily in connection with involuntary organ functions.

Node. An accumulation of cells; in connection with the heart, parts of the conducting system (atrioventricular node, sino-atrial node).

Oblique. Slanting; term used in X-ray technique to connote intermediate degrees of rotation of the body between front-back and side-to-side.

Occlusion. Blockage of the passage of blood in a blood vessel, usually caused by an obstacle inside the vessel.

Output, cardiac. The quantity of blood ejected by either cardiac ventricle.

Overload (pertaining to the heart). Increased work to be performed by the heart.

Oxygen consumption. Amount of oxygen used by a person in one minute to operate his body processes; its index is the amount of oxygen extracted from the air in one minute.

Pacemaker. A generator of rhythmic impulses causing cardiac contraction.

Pancarditis. Inflammatory disease of the heart involving all its three layers; same as "carditis."

Papillary muscle. Muscular column in a ventricle of the heart to which valves are attached through chordae tendineae.

Paroxysm. Sudden attack. *Paroxysmal*, appearing in episodes rather than continuously (e.g., paroxysmal dyspnea, paroxysmal tachycardia).

Periarteritis. Inflammatory disease of the smaller arteries extending into adjacent tissue around the arteries.

Pericardiocentesis. The procedure of removing fluid accumulated in the pericardial sac.

Pericarditis. Inflammatory disease of the pericardium.

Pericardium. Outer coating of the heart, consisting of two layers, the inner one firmly attached to the heart (epicardium) and the outer one forming a loose sac (parietal pericardium).

Petechiae. Small red spots caused by rupture of minute blood vessels.

Pheochromocytoma. Relatively rare tumor originating in the adrenal gland tissue, which produces an excess of hormones, causing high blood pressure and other disturbances of body function.

Phlebothrombosis. The formation of clots inside the vein without producing inflammatory reaction.

Phonocardiogram. A recording of heart sounds and murmurs.

Pleura. The membrane lining the lungs.

Polyarthritis. Inflammation of several body joints, either simultaneously or consecutively; a characteristic manifestation of rheumatic fever.

Postural. Pertaining to body posture. *Postural hypotension*, excessive fall in blood pressure caused by change from a recumbent to a standing position.

Prothrombin. A protein substance in the blood plasma involved in clot formation. *Prothrombin time*, blood test designed to assess the efficiency of the blood clotting process.

Pulmonary. Pertaining to the lungs or to circulation through the lungs.

Pulse. A wave of distention of the wall of a blood vessel coincidental with each heartbeat.

Pyelonephritis. Inflammatory disease of the kidney originating in its urine-collecting system.

Radiography. Examination of the body by means of X rays using photography on film.

Repolarization. The process of recharging heart muscle cells with electricity occurring during the relaxation period of the cardiac cycle.

Renal. Pertaining to the kidneys.

Retinopathy. Disease of the membrane lining the back part of the eye, especially common in severe hypertension.

Sarcoidosis. A chronic disease of unknown origin characterized by the formation of small nodules in various organs, including the heart.

Scleroderma. A chronic disease affecting the deeper layer of the skin and producing loss of elasticity of the skin; internal organs, including the heart, may also be involved.

Sedimentation rate. A blood test determining the speed with which red blood cells settle in a test tube, and related to the distribution of serum proteins.

Semilunar valves. Either of the two outflow valves of the heart, the pulmonary valve or aortic valve, characterized by three crescent-shaped leaflets.

Septum, cardiac. Partition between the two sides of the heart: *atrial septum*, between the atria; *ventricular septum*, between the ventricles.

Shunt. Passage of blood through abnormal communications between the two sides of the heart or between the aorta and the pulmonary artery.

Sign. Abnormality detected objectively by the physician in disease (in contrast to "symptom").

Sinoatrial node. Uppermost part of the cardiac conducting system—the normally active pacemaker of the heart.

Stenosis. Narrowing of the diameter of any structure, e.g., a cardiac orifice or a blood vessel.

Streptococcus. A microorganism responsible for many human diseases, particularly sore throats. In heart disease two strains are important: *hemolytic streptococcus*, to which rheumatic fever is related; *Streptococcus viridans*, which commonly produces bacterial endocarditis.

Stroke volume. The quantity of blood ejected by each ventricle in a single contraction.

Supraventricular. When pertaining to rhythm, abnormal mechanism of heartbeat originating in the atrium or the atrioventricular node.

Symptom. Subjective evidence of disease felt or observed by the patient.

Syncope. Sudden loss of consciousness.

Syndrome. A group of symptoms and signs occurring together, but not as well defined as a disease.

Systemic circulation. The larger of the two circuits involving the blood ejected by the left ventricle and returning to the right atrium, as opposed to pulmonary circulation.

Systemic lupus erythematosus. A chronic disease of the skin frequently invading internal organs, including the heart and blood vessels.

Systole. A stage of the cardiac cycle: muscular contraction.

Tachycardia. Rapid heartbeat, usually defined as above the rate of 100 beats per minute.

Tetralogy of Fallot. A congenital malformation of the heart characterized by a defect in the ventricular septum and obstruction to the outflow of blood from the right ventricle.

Therapy. Treatment.

Thromboangiitis. Inflammatory disease of the blood vessels associated with thrombus formation.

Thromboembolism. Intravascular clot formation associated with the transportation of clots by the bloodstream to distant parts of the body.

Thrombophlebitis. Clot formation in a vein with inflammation of the vein wall and surrounding tissue.

Thrombosis. The process of intravascular clot formation.

Thrombus. Clot formed inside a blood vessel.

Toxemia of pregnancy. Disease of unknown cause occurring during pregnancy and characterized by excessive retention of body fluids and high blood pressure.

Tricuspid. Pertaining to the valve separating the right atrium from the right ventricle.

Vectorcardiography. Graphic registration of the electric potential of the heart generated during heart action and differing from electrocardiography in that spatial orientation of the electric forces is registered.

Vein. A thin-walled blood vessel in which blood returns under low pressure from various parts of the body to the heart.

Vena cava. One of the two large veins (superior and inferior) returning venous blood to the right side of the heart.

Ventricle. One of two thick-walled muscular lower chambers of the heart which perform its principal pumping action.

Index